SAVING GRANDPA BILL

CHANGING YOUR LIFE BY CHANGING YOUR MIND

WILLIE "BILL" DAVIS

The Brand New Me ™
1098 Ann Arbor Road W STE 536
Plymouth, MI 48170
savinggrandpabill@gmail.com

All Scripture references are from the King James Version (KJV) of the Bible.

Published By: The Brand New Me
Cover Design: Bryan R. Martin (www.bryanrmartin.com)
Creative Storytelling: Kimberly Ratliff (www.kreneecreative.com)
Project Consultant: Shaun Maloy (www.maloyfamily.com)

ISBN: 979-8-9890761-3-0 (Paperback)
ISBN: 979-8-9890761-4-7 (Hardback)
ISBN: 979-8-9890761-5-4 (E-book)

PRAISE FOR SAVING GRANDPA BILL

Every young person who enters the field of medicine will very likely tell you that they did so because of a love for science and a desire to help people. Medicine is in large part the practical application of science to improve the quality and longevity of human life. The acquisition of a knowledge base and set of skills to carry out this work is arduous and lifelong. The requirements of study and practice can produce highly skilled individuals capable of miraculous interventions that ease suffering and disease.

While we are helping people, sometimes the focus needed to treat a problem before us can make the most well-intentioned physician myopic. We hear and see the person before us but only in part. There are occasions, however, where our efforts produce something that is uplifting, not only to our patients but to us as well. Sometimes the result is bigger than what we have done as a physician.

This is a story that tells of one of those occasions. It is a therapeutic relationship where both physician and patient are left better because of an interaction. A story of a few words and a plan bringing life-altering changes. It is the best that a patient and a doctor can achieve. It is a reminder to physicians that when we become myopic from the challenges of our profession, we need to remember something. In our best moments we do not treat disease or suffering.

In our best moments we touch someone's life,
and they touch ours.

That is the true destination of a therapeutic relationship. This is a story of what can be done when facing a challenge. It is a story that can surely be therapeutic for you as well.

William Higginbotham III MD, FAAOS, FACS

Thank you, my beautiful wife, Denise, for being by
my side and supporting me throughout the years.
You are the love of my life, and I thank you for loving
me through thin and thick and now thin again.

Thank you to my children and grandchildren for motivating
me and giving me a legacy to behold. I want to witness
all that life offers and all God will do through you!

Thank you to Jeff Taylor Jr. (RIH), Marcus Haynes, Robert
Compton, and Matt Mckoy for your day one support and
encouragement. Also, to my superstar fitness crew for cheering
me on (you know who you are). There is nothing like having
friends along this path who will sweat and celebrate the
milestones with you!

Thank You Kimberly Ratcliff and the K. Renee Creative Agency,
Shaun Maloy and Maloy Family Books, and thank you
Bryan R. Martin for helping this book become a reality.
May our successes be many in service to the one who created us.

CONTENTS

Foreword xi

Introduction xvii

Chapter One   A Few Things to Consider 1

Chapter Two   Losing Grandpa Bill..13

Chapter Three   The Mentality of Obesity....................................23

Chapter Four   Conversations with Myself 33

Chapter Five   The Journey...43

Chapter Six   The Brand New Me..59

Chapter Seven   Moving Forward...69

Conclusion...77

About The Author 87

FOREWORD

Know ye not that ye are the temple of God, and that the Spirit of God dwelleth in you?

—I Corinthians 3:16

One of the most extraordinary things the Lord God gifted all mankind with was the power of choice. I get excited just thinking about it; out of all the ways that lie before us, we have the power to choose which path we will take. We do not have to wait for life to happen. We can make it happen.

That's what Willie Davis did; he made something happen. From a physical standpoint, he'd allowed his life to fall into disrepair to the point that it threatened his very existence. Although he could have blamed it on his upbringing, his metabolism, or even depression, any excuse could have landed him squarely over four hundred pounds. But the good news is that he decided to do something about it. That is the inspiration in his story, and it can be the inspiration in your story. You may not have a weight problem, but whatever obstacle you may be facing in your life, you have the power to change it!

I have known Willie Davis for many years and have had a front-row seat to his transformation. I saw his initial victory firsthand, only to watch him fall back into those same habits and regain all the weight he had lost. He could have stopped at that point and concluded that it was just his lot to be big. But he had a better vision for himself, which included being better for his wife and children, and ultimately, his future. He chose to make a change because he saw himself differently than what he saw in the mirror. He did something that only he could do. He transformed his life by renewing his mind.

I remember him telling me how good a basketball player he was and how he would ball with my younger brother Daniel. I could not see it because the Willie that I was looking at was far different from that Willie of his past.

I want you to examine your life, and if it does not measure up to the life you have envisioned for yourself, then read this book, answer the questions in the workbook, and take charge of you.

We have been created to inspire and help others through our personal journeys. To do that, you must take control of your life as Willie Davis did. As you read this book, I am confident it will resonate with you as it did with me. This book is transformative and will give you ideas to help you achieve all the plans you have laid out for your life.

Thank you, brother Willie Davis, for sharing your ups and downs, your ebbs and flows, and your tragedies and triumphs so that we might attain the best that God has for us.

—Bishop Marvin L. Winans Sr.
Grammy Award Winning Gospel Singer, Songwriter, and Founder/Pastor of Perfecting Church

After co-founding the Powerhouse Gym and spending decades in the fitness business, some might assume I've seen every wonder there is to see in the health and fitness world. I've worked with countless individuals in the health and wellness industry and have seen plenty of awe-inspiring weight loss journeys and body transformations. While there are many ways to take control of your health and reclaim your life, I have always enjoyed witnessing the results of hard work and dedication!

It was like a breath of fresh air to meet Willie Davis and witness his amazing transformation. The thing that sets this man apart from the rest is how he was able to accomplish this impressive feat at the age of sixty-eight. Of course, I've watched people in their twenties and thirties turn their lives around. Seeing this at his age is mind-blowing! When this man needed to lose over two hundred pounds to be fit enough for a hip replacement and heal his body, he made the decision and got it done!

To see the mental fortitude and commitment and watching him connect with and positively influence so many others along the way, was the making of a fitness legend. It has genuinely been my immense pleasure to know him and have him as a part of my gym family.

When I say that this book is just the beginning of the impact his story will have on the world, trust me, and know that you can benefit greatly from reading this book and riding the wave of motivation and encouragement that he creates in his wake. I see how he inspires those around him to push harder and go farther, so let that same life-changing energy propel you to the best life you can dream of and beyond.

You've got this! We'll see you on the other side!

—Will Dabish
Cofounder, President, and CEO
Powerhouse Gyms International

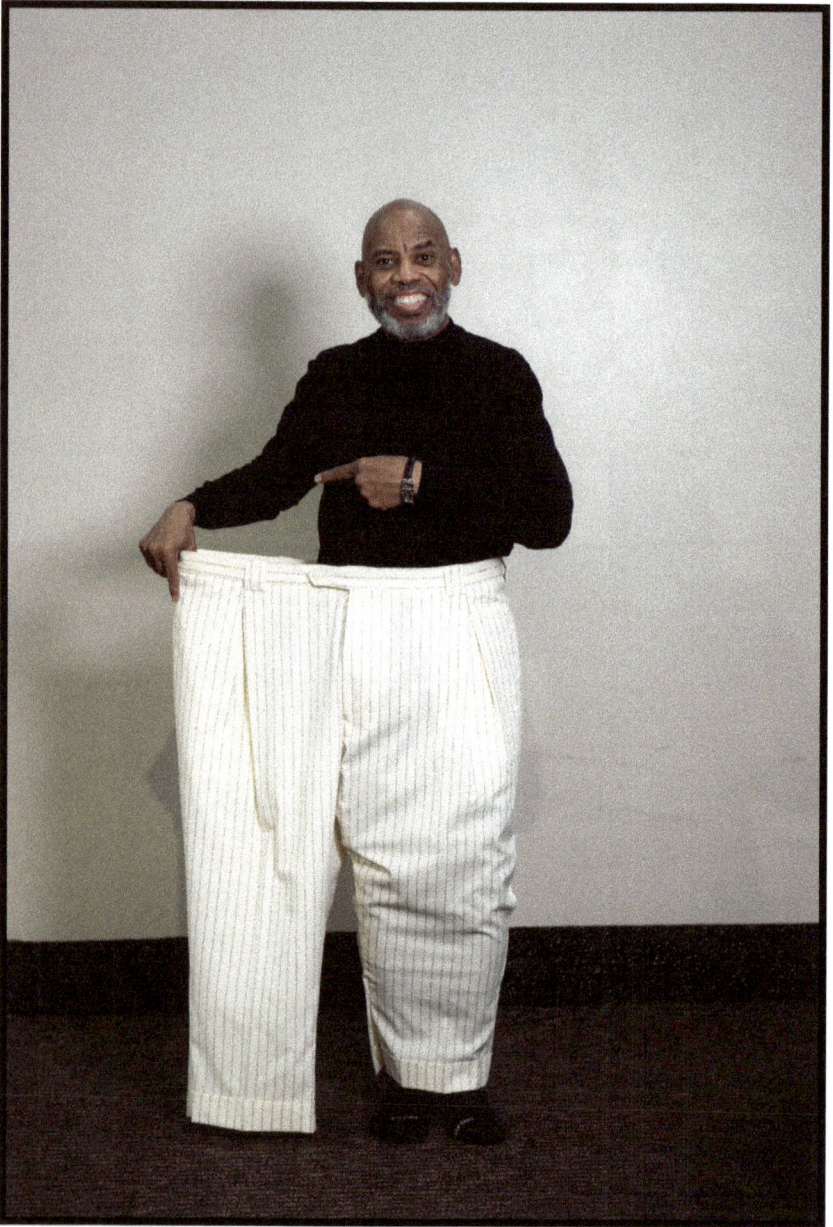

INTRODUCTION

Hey, superstar! You might be staring at this page as a last-ditch effort to motivate yourself to change your life, or maybe you've never even tried to make a change before. Either way, I'm glad you're here! I'm happy because I want you to add years of fulfilling life to your story, and there is no better way to do that than to get your health in order.

Our bodies are just like the machines we create. When they're well maintained and treated with care, they last longer and perform better as they were designed. On the flip side, when our bodies are misused, and no maintenance is performed, they break down. If you're tired of the unpleasant process of premature breakdown, then you grabbed the right book. The best news I have for you is that you can start performing excellent self-care and maintenance today! If you're still living, you can take steps to improve. Tackling your physical health is a great starting point!

However, my journey has also shown me that there is much more to a quality life than good physical fitness. Life is far more meaningful when you feel good and maintain excellent health

HEALTH IS THE GREATEST OF HUMAN BLESSINGS.
—Hippocrates

physically, mentally, emotionally, and spiritually. All these aspects work together for holistic health and wealth. In this book, I share how I've changed my physical health as well as the health of every other part of who I am. I simply didn't want to look fantastic and live longer; I wanted to be great. I want to enjoy the rest of my life and inspire others to do the same.

When people run into me now, they often express shock and awe at who they see in front of them. Let's be real; when you lose two hundred pounds, you become a new person on the outside. Still, I want you to understand that the transformation that I experienced on the inside was far more necessary than what you see on the outside. That's the journey I want to help you begin. And listen, I call you superstar because I know you can do this. I know that you can tap into the supernatural power within to catalyze a life-changing transformation. You can realize the life that you're meant to enjoy. Read it, believe it, and act like it, superstar!

So many aspects of my thought processes, eating habits, life rhythms, and spiritual awareness needed to change. And to make those changes and actually stick to them, I needed to know why I was committing to the changes and why that commitment was nonnegotiable. So let me share a few things I realized.

When you have a why you will never have to worry about the how. The why will look different for each person. I can't determine your why, but if you don't already know your why, maybe mine will make you consider your circumstances differently. A few conclusions I came to motivated me to make a change.

I was tired.

At almost four hundred pounds, I finally woke up after stepping on my special scale that could register more than 350 pounds. Contrary to popular belief, approaching four hundred pounds is no easy feat for someone like me. It took decades of yo-yo dieting and slowly adding X after X to my large-sized clothing. Finally, I found myself in fewer and fewer pictures and filled my life with busyness that got a lot of good things done but left my health on the back burner. The journey to obesity takes many twists and turns, but it can sneak up on you.

Convenience became the name of the game so that I could work longer hours. Convenience also allowed me to be a leader at my church, support my wife's entrepreneurial pursuits, and provide the suburban lifestyle for my family. In my mind, it helped me ensure that my children and grandchildren could achieve things that the generations before them had not.

By the time I decided to change my story, I was tired. I was tired of carrying the extra weight. I was tired of taking multiple medications for various health issues. I was tired of not liking what I saw when I slowed down enough to look in the mirror. I was tired of accommodating the extra space my body took up in the world.

I was just tired.

I decided my family deserved to have me around.

My wife, children, and grandchildren love me, and they want to have as much time as possible with me. So, I have to give them as much time as possible. Living a healthy life is paramount to making that happen. I have eleven grandchildren who want to have plenty of memories of our time together when I'm gone. Not only that, but I want to see my grandchildren hit every milestone in their lives. I want to see them graduate from high school and college. I want to witness marriages and become Great-Grandpa Bill.

I finally decided that how I treat myself impacts more than just me. It dramatically affects my family for generations to come. I started this journey at close to seventy years old, so I hope to inspire you to start now and reclaim your time. Your family will thank you!

I still have an impact to make.

Since I'm not just living for myself, I know that my life impacts others. Every one of us has an impact to make. I've watched younger people than me deal with similar health issues and succumb to complications. My younger brother died before me, and I was heavier than him and dealing with the same health issues. I've often marveled at still being here because I know it could have easily been me. I do not take it lightly that I'm still here. Since beginning this journey, I've connected with so many people with extraordinary stories and even more who are on the precipice of their own transformative journey.

It has become abundantly clear that there is important work left for me to do. What's more, I've come to realize that I'll have a better time doing that work if I keep myself in the best health possible. So, if you're reading this, it means you still have work to do that will send ripples out to change the lives of countless others.

Don't take the importance of your life lightly. Once you realize there is work of magnitude to be done and you're the only one who can do it, committing to the changes you need to make to reclaim your time is a no-brainer. You can do this!

One more thing …

Throughout this book, you'll find the steps I used to make the change, but I want you to think of this less as a step-by-step guide and more as a companion. My purpose in sharing my story is to show you that anyone can make the necessary changes to have the quality of life that we're supposed to have. There is no cookie-cutter recipe for this type of transformation, though. Hopefully, this book will help you figure out the unique steps you need to take to change your life. I've included reflection prompts, workout, and meal-planning ideas, and more to inspire your journey.

It's time to become the new you, superstar! But, before we get started, take some time, and answer these questions.

What is the most significant health concern you currently have?

_____

_____

_____

_____

What is your ultimate health goal?

_____

_____

_____

_____

What is your most pressing obstacle to getting healthy?

_____

_____

_____

_____

DIET GOES FAR BEYOND WHAT YOU EAT.

YOU NEED TO CHANGE THE DIET OF YOUR MIND.

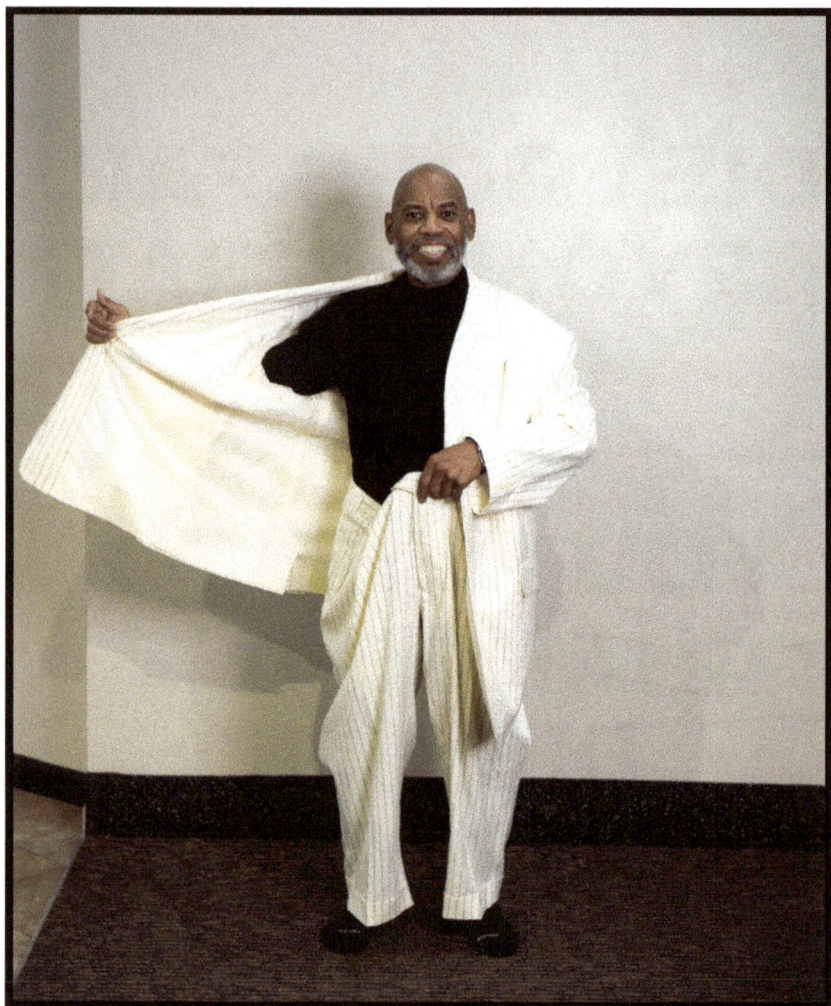

CHAPTER ONE

A FEW THINGS TO CONSIDER

O K, superstar! Before we get started, you need to understand this: You don't get close to four hundred pounds overnight. And you can't heal your mind and body overnight either.

I'd love to tell you there was some magic pill or trick that helped me get motivated, move, and drop pounds, but there wasn't. My journey to the new me took discipline, perseverance, grit, and more than a little good humor. I found people to help me when I needed direction or encouragement. Still, ultimately, I had to change the way I thought about food, myself, and the value of my life. I had to prioritize my health.

The single most significant change that has taken place throughout my health journey is my mindset. The only way I could make the changes I needed and consistently show up for myself and my family was to change the fundamental building blocks of my thinking. I can assure you that was no small feat, because I'd been conditioned to think in specific patterns by my culture, my circle of influence, and society. The truth is that if we allow ourselves to accept the status quo of our society, we will often be less healthy, whole, and happy as a result.

LIVING A HEALTHY LIFESTYLE WILL ALWAYS BE A PERSONAL DECISION FOR EVERYONE, BUT WE CAN ALWAYS PASS THE MESSAGE TO THOSE WHO NEED THE HELP.
—Odeta Rose

I had to get honest about the things that were enabling me to continue the course of self-destruction and reprogram my commitment to them. When I finally faced reality, I discovered that many seemingly innocuous actions sabotage our efforts to live life to our fullest potential. These seemingly harmless actions keep us from creating the legacy we want to leave behind.

What we consume has so much more to do with how we show up in this world than we realize. I've found one of my life's assignments is to pull back the curtain.

At sixty-eight years old, if I could change my entire life and inspire those around me to do the same, you can certainly do it too. There is no limit to the richness of time you can reclaim if you examine your life, change your thinking, and stay the course. You've got this, superstar!

Let's get started.

The battle is in the mind.

"As a man thinketh in his heart, so is he."

--Proverbs 23:7

It's no secret the mind is a powerful thing. Both religion and science have discovered numerous indications that the brain is both powerful and complex beyond what we even understand. Beyond single-handedly orchestrating the function of the human body, the human mind has been the originator of all of humanity's inventions and imaginings. The medical field is awash with accounts of the power of the mind as a healing mechanism beyond explanation. We now understand that our mindset can change everything from our mood to the trajectory of our lives.

There is much truth in the statement that your mindset dictates your reality. So that's where we'll start.

There is power in what you believe to be true.

I'm sure you've heard the story of the emperor's new clothes, right? Just to refresh your memory, I'll recap. The story revolves around a ruler who loves to wear the best and latest designs. He spends all his time and money focusing on that instead of his other responsibilities. So, when two wise guys roll into town and promise the latest in fashion—magnificent clothing invisible to fools—he jumps on it. They make a show of setting up their work tools, and whenever the ruler or his advisers visit, they all pretend to see the clothes because they don't want to seem like fools. Then when the clothes are "ready," the crooks pretend to dress him, and the ruler goes to appear in a parade. Not wanting to be labeled fools, his subjects pretend to see the clothes, too, until a child proclaims that the ruler isn't wearing anything.

I bring up that fable to illustrate what the tale itself reveals. We will do just about anything if it aligns with what we have forced ourselves to believe. Most of us will deny the possibility of being swindled by outside forces or other people that we would do something like leave our homes completely naked. Still, if you think about it, we unfortunately do things like this every day. We allow our crazy schedules to convince us it's OK to eat food that's horrible for our bodies. We convince ourselves that sleeping less than we need is fine if we're chasing unrealistic deadlines. We cut out the physical activity we need in favor of commuting for a position with a higher salary. At some point, we must realize that believing so many of these lies is keeping us from realizing how we're meant to live.

At the risk of getting too deep, I must ask you to consider the sum of your life thus far. Are you pleased with what your life has become in every area, from your physical health to your spiritual health? If not, now is the time to change that. Now is the time to reclaim your wealth.

Your health is the wealth of the heart, mind, body, and soul.

I'd love to say I've spent most of my life building wealth in my heart, mind, body, and soul just as much as in my bank account. While I have paid particular attention to my soul's health and wealth, my body was probably the last thing on the list most of the time. When I was young, I looked good. I was an athlete. I was never overweight. After high school, other things took more priority. The truth is that I spent decades building the American

4

dream for my family and taking care of myself got pushed to the bottom of the list.

Listen, I'm a black man born and raised in Detroit, Michigan. When I was growing up, no one in my circle of influence talked about health and fitness as much as they dreamed about making it out of the hood. Most people were doing something phenomenal if they graduated from high school and got a good job working in one of the automotive factories.

I grew up watching my parents make a life for us with partial high school educations. My father worked two jobs to provide for us. He was always going and was very physically active in his employment. He looked good and fit on the outside, but his eating habits left much to be desired. We were on the typical diet of fried foods, starches, and grease. We ate vegetables, but most of the time they were flavored with fat and pork. Cleaning up our eating habits just wasn't on the agenda. It wasn't even on the radar. We just liked to eat food that tasted good! I still do.

It wasn't just at home, either. The same was true of church and social gatherings. You know how it goes. If someone got married, had a birthday, or passed away, the meal was anchored with fried chicken and pork chops, ham, or ribs, depending on the season. In addition to the rich and often fatty meats, the cooks made savory soul food sides, and they never failed to bake sugary sweet cakes, pies, and puddings. I grew up among some of the best cooks Detroit has ever seen. You can't tell me any differently. They really gave a whole new meaning to the phrase "comfort food." So, it's no wonder that my fit-on-the-outside father suffered a stroke during a procedure to clean up his arteries. He dealt with the complications of that stroke for the rest of his life. But it would be decades before I made the connection that what's going in and happening inside my body is just as important as how I look on the outside and how physically active, I was.

During my decades of gaining a whole additional person's worth of weight, no one told me I was doing anything wrong. I think that was because I built the picture-perfect life for myself and my family. Even though I only had a high school diploma, I had a great career. I was able to move my family to the suburbs of Detroit and provide a life for them that centered around faith, education, personal improvement, community leadership, and the American dream. We could afford nice things, travel, and give to those in need. It was important to me that my daughters were well educated and could provide for themselves, never needing to rely on a man to take care of them. My children deserved to have every opportunity this life afforded them. I think I did a pretty good job, but it came at the expense of my health.

I spent my days working long hours, fulfilling the leadership responsibilities in my church, and going to my children's games and recitals now and again. In the shuffle of all that, I just sort of lost sight of myself. As the size of my clothing got larger and larger, I simply found myself in front of fewer and fewer cameras. Not once did a trusted friend, coworker, or church leader pull me to the side and encourage me to take inventory of my holistic health. While I was morbidly obese, no one directly communicated the fear that I was shortening my lifespan. People may have given me side-eye when I walked on the airplane, but no one addressed the elephant in the room.

The fact is that most Americans are equally blind to anything outside of the pursuit of success. The cost of that pursuit on our health, relationships, and life in general simply goes ignored. The latest statistics from the Centers for Disease Control and Prevention say more than 70 percent of Americans aged twenty and over at overweight, and more than 40 percent are obese. That's a problem!

When you consider all the health issues that arise due to obesity, these numbers are staggering and saddening. Think of all the lives lost because folks don't have the information and resources to get healthier, or they just don't think they have what it takes to change their lives.

When I finally found myself mourning the loss of my younger brother from complications of diabetes and hypertension, I was closer to four hundred pounds than three hundred. I was suffering from deteriorating health and quality of life, and it just clicked. I needed to make a change.

Remember that special scale I mentioned stepping on in the introduction? It registered my weight at 368 pounds. I felt like I was one sandwich away from four hundred pounds. So, I looked in the mirror and asked myself, "What about some form of weight loss surgery? I immediately said to myself, "Nah, man; I'm not doing surgery. It didn't take any surgery to gain the weight". That was the moment I concocted the plan to change my life forever. That was it. That was the moment my journey began.

How is your holistic health today?

_____

_____

_____

_____

How do you currently think about diet and fitness?

_____

_____

_____

_____

What areas have taken priority in your life?

_____

_____

_____

_____

ADDITIONAL NOTES:

_____

_____

_____

_____

_____

_____

_____

_____

_____

_____

_____

_____

_____

THE WORST
LIES ARE THE
ONES YOU
TELL YOURSELF
ABOUT THE
WAY YOU LOOK
AND FEEL.

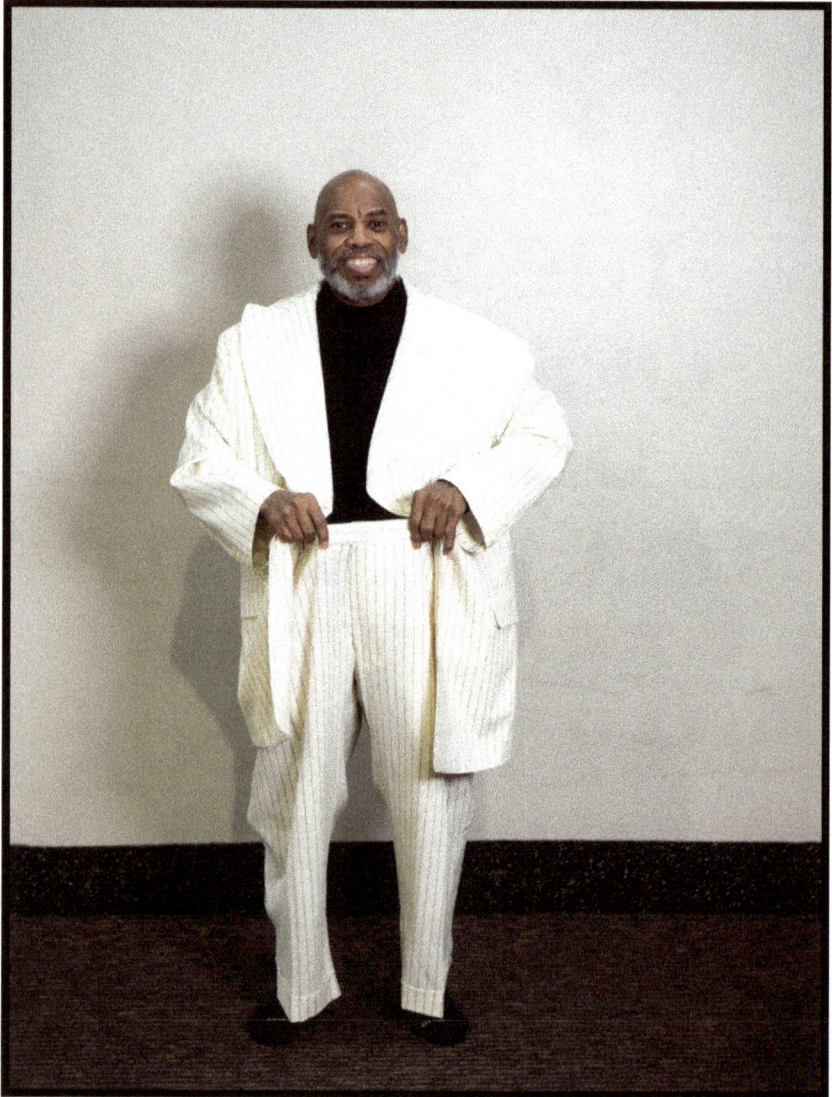

CHAPTER TWO

LOSING GRANDPA BILL

When I was growing up, I didn't know either grandfather. They had passed on, so my elders were my loving grandmother, my parents, and a host of uncles and aunts. At the time, it was just my reality. I never really thought much about the absence of my grandfathers, but as I got older, it started to be on my mind more and more.

As I got closer to the age of having grandchildren, I began to consider my frailty. I thought about the possible impact of not having living grandfathers on a child. You have a limited understanding of where you come from and the importance of firsthand multigenerational familial relationships when your family has only had two living generations for most of your lifetime. There is a richness in sitting and talking with your grandparents, great-grandparents, and beyond.

I found myself wanting to change the experience of my family. I wanted my grandchildren to have me for years to come. I wanted to share my personal experiences with them, including what I've learned about healthy living. I wanted to see them graduate from college and get married. I wanted to meet my great-grandchildren and for them to feel the impact of having four living generations.

As this desire increasingly filled my heart, I realized every poor health decision was shortening my days and stealing that experience from my legacy. So, I decided to move in reverse and reclaim my time. I'd decided what to do, but it took some doing to figure out and commit to how I'd do it. I think I'm getting a little ahead of myself, though. So, before I go on, let me backtrack. This journey began long before I made this decision to lengthen my life. It really started before I had any apparent health and weight issues.

It goes without saying that no one gains hundreds of pounds overnight. The truth of weight gain and loss is it's easier to gain weight than lose it, in most cases. It's the funniest thing. Some people in your family or close circle may comment on your appearance when you're getting wider, but we're more likely to engage in a silent commentary as a society. We'll talk to others about someone's weight, but only the boldest members of society address it directly with the one packing on the pounds. Don't get me wrong; there is never a place for shaming those who don't fit into conventional norms of body type and weight, but sometimes people need a little wake-up call in the health department. In all the years that I struggled with my weight, who knows how much sooner I would have turned it around had someone I loved and respected pulled me aside and told me the truth about the way I was shortening my life by failing to address the elephant in my room.

It took time for me to get to where I was when I finally made a fundamental change. As I mentioned before, I wasn't always overweight. As a child and young adult, I looked good! OK? There was a lot that went into making me an obese sixty-eight-year-old. My parents did the best they knew how, and I did too. The truth is that I was, in many ways, ignorant of all the things that were affecting the way I thought, ate, and lived. I couldn't do better, with a lasting impact, until I knew better and transformed my mentality.

I can recall what life was like for me as a child just as vividly as if it was yesterday. My mother and father raised seven of us on the east side of Detroit in a three-bedroom house on Bewick Street. My mother was a sweet but strong homemaker. She had to be with six boys and one girl. She nurtured us, kept us in line, and fed us well! When I say well, I mean we had food that tasted good, and we never wasted what was on our plates. Many of you reading now have had a parent or grandparent implore you to finish all your food because there are starving children somewhere who wish they had just a fraction of what you had. Our portion control was whatever portion was presented to us. Being full meant a clean plate, and therein lies the beginning of gluttony. We'll touch on that issue of gluttony later but suffice it to say I had no idea what eating healthy looked like, even though my body had yet to show visible signs.

Growing up, we had a typical urban family dynamic. My father worked six full days a week during his forty-year career at the Chrysler Corporation and worked a second job at Burton-Mercy Hospital. When he wasn't working, he fixed things for people around the neighborhood. He was a jack-of-all-trades, and my brothers and I were his helpers. He would take us when he went to work on someone's car or around their house, and we would do whatever he told us. It wasn't long before I got wise and got into sports because if I had a game on Saturday, I didn't have to go and work with my dad. I was already interested in sports anyway, but now I had an excuse to avoid long hours working with my father and brothers. Turns out I was a much better-than-average ballplayer! I ended up playing football, basketball, and baseball.

So, I was in good shape all through my teens and twenties. I weighed less than 175 pounds when I first met my wife in 1978. The issue was not how I started; it was how I continued. After eating really well at my mother's table and burning all the calories on the court or field, I continued eating how I liked at my wife's table. The only change was my activity level. I slowed down. And I mean way down. The way life goes for many of us is just the same. We slow down, sit down, and fill out. Something to think about is whether your activity levels match your eating habits. Once you get that cushy office job and stop walking as much, does your body need the same number of calories to support the movement of your body? No.

I found that as life changed, I didn't take inventory of my diet, exercise level, and overall wellness. It was a slow creep, so as I found my clothes getting a little tighter, I just headed over to the store to purchase clothes with a different letter on the tag instead of looking at what lifestyle changes were needed. As we started having children and our calendar got even fuller, time became more of a commodity, and convenience became the name of the game. In my pursuit of a middle-class lifestyle, I lost sight of my well-being.

I overlooked the way I was neglecting my wellness because I was doing so well in the other areas of my life. So, the question is, what have you prioritized at the expense of your health?

THE FIRST WEALTH IS HEALTH.
—Ralph Waldo Emerson

Most folks in America want to be wealthy. We live in a society where the middle and upper-middle-class lifestyle is the goal. It's enough to be very comfortable, and it's within reach with an education or a good work ethic. So, when most people think about wealth, they think of the number of zeros in their bank account, among other material possessions. For me, the pursuit of that suburban lifestyle for my family became a focal point, alongside the growth and health of my soul. My definition of wealth needed to be transformed, though!

As I began to have a desire to leave a beautiful legacy with my children and future generations, I had to decide what my most valuable assets would be. Of course, my faith is always at the top of the list of values I wish to pass along to anyone I meet. So, that has always been at the forefront of my mind. I never wanted to leave this world the same way I entered it, superstar. I have always wanted to have an impact.

I've come to understand that the impact I make and the legacy I leave to future generations needs to be more than financial. I need to leave a legacy of knowledge that there is more to life than what we have. We can do so much for those around us if we are in optimal health. There is a richness in taking care of your body so that you can live life to the fullest and be here to fulfill your life's purpose far longer than if you sit on the couch and eat yourself into an early grave.

Your health is truly the first wealth you should pursue and maintain. If you fail to do that, you'll only experience life at half capacity, and that's a sad existence, indeed. So, let's take inventory of what your current focus is.

If today was your last day on earth, what would your legacy be?

_____

_____

_____

_____

What areas of your life do you need to reprioritize to improve your quality of life?

_____

_____

_____

_____

What is your current go-to indicator for your level of healthiness?

_____

_____

_____

_____

ADDITIONAL NOTES:

EVERY GOAL WILL HAVE A MYRIAD OF CHALLENGES.

OVERCOME THEM ALL!

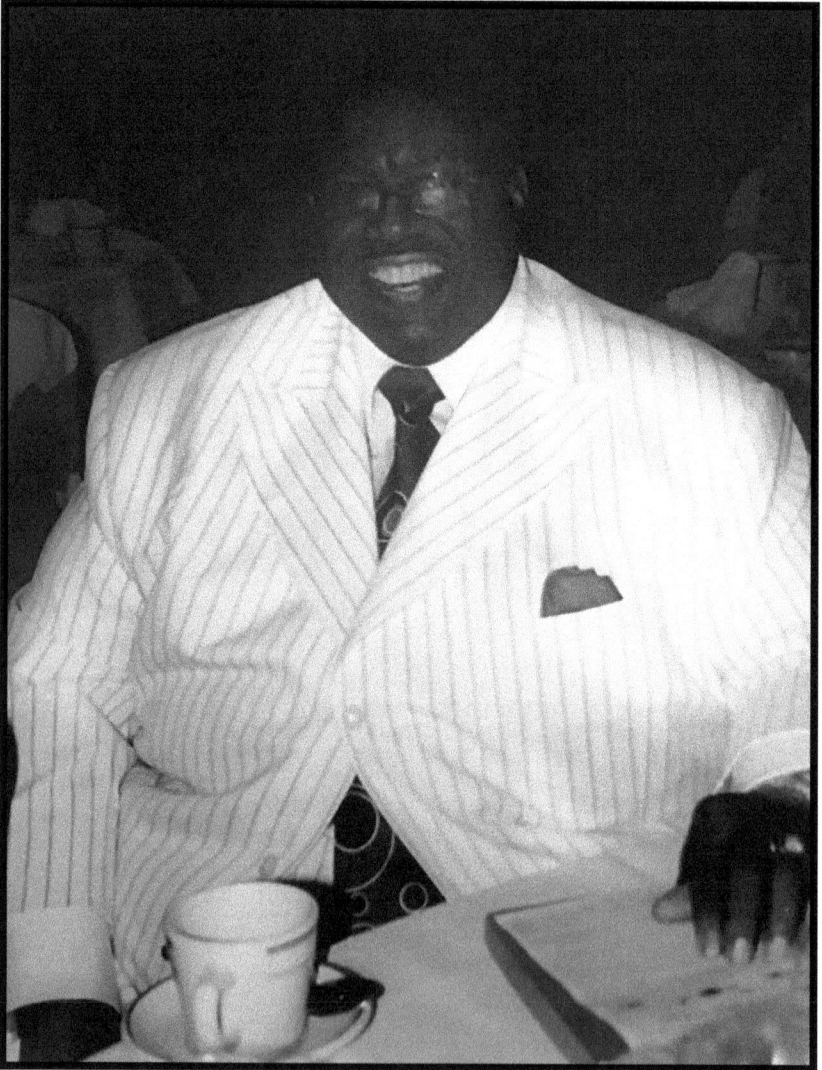

CHAPTER THREE

THE MENTALITY OF OBESITY

t's the oddest thing. As I've mentioned, I can't remember a single instance of being directly or indirectly told that I need to drop this weight. I went decades having the conscious and unconscious existence of someone growing increasingly obese, but not one medical professional, leader, mentor at work or church, or family member sat me down to have that much-needed intervention conversation about my health.

When I think back, it seems as if every aspect of our modern American culture has conspired against me being in good health while it has mocked me as I gained pound after pound. I've been acutely aware of the inconveniences that arise when you can't fit into the "normal"-sized space that we, as a society, have allotted for each person. I know what it's like to have to buy larger shoes, not because my foot is longer, but because it's wider than it should be. I've lamented not being able to use regular towels because they don't wrap fully around my frame. And let's not even get into the wholly uncomfortable experience of trying to travel by plane.

There is a silent shame in asking for a safety belt extender. I've found that timing is of the utmost importance in this situation because you don't want to hold everything up once everyone has boarded and the attendants start doing the safety checks. So, you must remember to discreetly ask for the extender before you sit down so that you can be ready once the cabin is in the final check before takeoff. Say amen, somebody.

I have many insights to share about the mindset that being obese puts you in, but before I continue, let's review a few facts about obesity, just to put things in perspective.

THE WAY TO DEAL WITH THE DEVIL OF OBESITY AND DIABETES IS LITERALLY ONE DAY AT A TIME.

—Stephen Furst

In general, obesity is classified as having a body weight higher than what is considered healthy for a given height. The medical tool most often used to screen for obesity is the body mass index or BMI. Now, if you know anything about anthropology and the diversity of body compositions, you know that using the BMI alone doesn't always give an accurate picture of an individual's fitness level. Still, it's a tool that can be used to approximate how much you should weigh.

BMI is calculated by dividing a person's weight in kilograms by the square of their height, in meters. Often, a high BMI indicates a high level of body fat.

When you do this calculation, a BMI between eighteen and a

half and twenty-five is generally accepted as healthy, with a BMI ranging from twenty-five to thirty putting you in the overweight category. Higher than thirty is considered obese. There are additional levels as the number gets higher and higher, with over forty being categorized as severely obese, in most cases.

The medical risks of being obese are numerous and well documented, and since so many Americans fall into that category, there is a genuine concern in the medical field.

Children and adults alike are being affected by more and more health problems because of their weight. And while there are medical conditions that can cause weight gain, most people who struggle with obesity do so because they're overeating, eating the wrong foods, and often eating too late in the evening.

In the last chapter, I mentioned the word gluttony, and if I'm honest with you, America has a culture of gluttony. If you're not familiar with this concept, it is generally understood as an issue with excessive eating and drinking.

So, that's clearly part of what has led to the obesity issue that we face as a country, but the spirit of gluttony is something else entirely. The compulsion to excessively consume often reaches far past food and drink. It can become a habit to excessively consume anything our whims turn to. When this issue goes unchecked, it leaves any care for health and wellness behind; it can even hurt our wallets just as much, if not more, than it hurts our expanding waistbands.

The mentality of gluttony compels us to consume until we're past full, but the trick of the ever-expanding belly and appetite is that when we push ourselves to consume everything we see, we force our capacity to grow. So, we end up forever consuming more than we should. That's why the habit of cleaning your plate works against your health goals.

It's OK to leave food on the plate if you've satisfied your nutritional needs and you feel satisfied. After a while, your eyes will learn what portions are necessary, and your meals will grow smaller and more colorful, with leafy greens, colorful vegetables, and fruits. As you take time to eat mindfully, you'll be able to more accurately gauge when you are feeling satisfied instead of stuffed full.

So, it was for me. Once I decided to escape the mentality of obesity and change my life, I had to fight to discipline my mind, body, and appetite. I could not eat with abandon at all times of day and night. Our bodies need time to digest what we eat. So, if you eat around the clock, your body never has time to process what has already been consumed and rest.

That's also another reason for many of the illnesses connected with obesity. Those health issues literally start in the gut. If you heal your mentality around food and treat your body well, you can also heal many of your physical ailments!

Beyond the physical benefits, I've found that losing all that extra weight I was carrying lifted the load of the mental and emotional weight I was carrying, too! Let's get real—there is an element of shame that comes with each new belt you must purchase, or the wardrobe tricks you have to use for your clothing to fit better. When you have to mentally consider the type of chair or couch you're about to sit on because you may have issues fitting or getting back up after you sit, it takes an emotional toll. Something as simple as picking things up off the floor becomes a huge undertaking once you're past a certain weight and you find that you can't move around as quickly or freely as you once did.

I remember thinking about whether a lawn chair or beach bed could hold my weight while vacationing. I'd often opt for a towel on the sand. The only issue with that was the rolling around and maneuvering I'd have to do to get up off the ground. That's not how we're supposed to live. We should be able to enjoy our time here as much as possible. We are supposed to have abundant life as we experience all God has created for us. There are so many aspects of being obese that drain the joy from everyday life. It's time to reclaim your joy and lengthen your time.

The truth is that obesity affects every aspect of your life, and though no one was directly telling me to make a change, folks have their ways of trying to nudge you in the right direction of losing weight. It's almost like polite society has an unconscious urge to silently comment on folks who are obese without having the tough-love conversation. When family and friends do this, it's counterproductive for many reasons. The first is that it is frustrating because it reinforces the mentality that you aren't in a good place without giving you the positive and direct support you need to make a lasting change.

Besides that, it also keeps us from engaging in one of the greatest gifts of life—open, transparent, and caring relationships. When we comment on issues generally as a society but fail to engage in those conversations on an interpersonal level with the ones we love and care about, we rob ourselves of authentic community and meaningful change as a society. Instead, everything is taboo. Many people are left alone, and they find it easier to ignore their issues rather than face them head-on and make a change.

So, with every additional ten to twenty pounds that I gained, I lost a part of who I was. Everyday life became much more complicated, but I did not have the time or space to do uncomplicated things. If I'm honest, I was in a sort of survival mode that was sabotaging my survival. In my relentless pursuit of a better life, I failed to live better. My thought patterns needed to shift from what was convenient and comfortable to what would help me make the necessary changes I needed to reclaim my best life.

What are some things you would look forward to doing if you lost weight?

_____

_____

_____

_____

What are some of the thought processes you've considered because of your excess weight?

_____

_____

_____

_____

How has your physical health affected your mental health?

_____

_____

_____

_____

ADDITIONAL NOTES:

BE HONEST WITH YOURSELF.

WHAT SIZE DO YOU WANT TO BE?

SAY IT OUT LOUD AND WORK TO GET THERE.

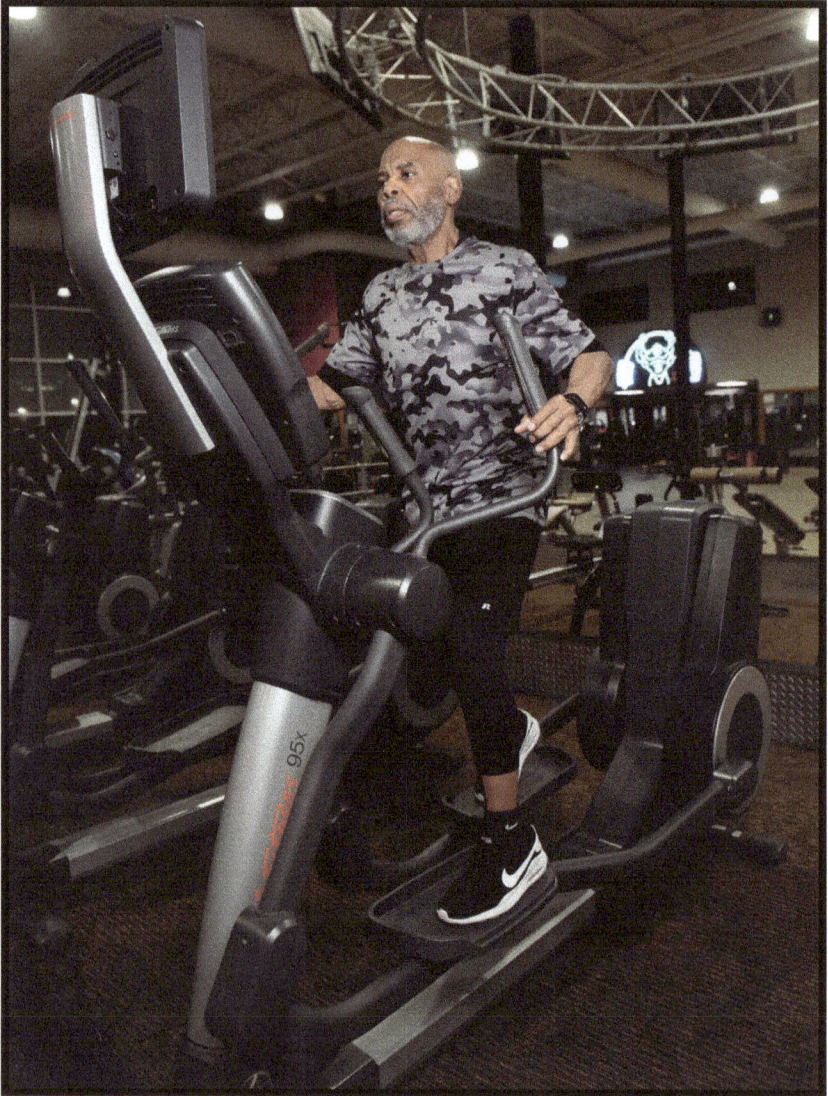

CHAPTER FOUR

CONVERSATIONS WITH MYSELF

Beloved, I wish above all things that thou mayest prosper and be in health, even as thy soul prospereth.

—3 John 1:2

O K, superstar, so how did I completely turn my life around? The answer is as simple as it is ongoing—I decided to choose God's best for myself. So, when I decided that I had to lose weight without going the surgical route, I needed to make several huge decisions. The first was to be real with myself.

I mentioned before that I had filled my life with overtime at work and leadership responsibilities at church. On top of that, I had a responsibility to my family, so my plate was full, literally, and figuratively. So, there's that unpleasant reality again—overconsumption. I needed to add margins to my life. I needed to make space to care for myself, make better health decisions, and focus on what was truly and urgently important.

After losing my father to complications a few years after a stroke brought on by bypass surgeries for clogged arteries and my brother to complications from obesity and diabetes, I was awakened to the dangers I was facing. The truth is, as a society we have a terrible habit of blaming big bones for the extra weight that we carry from generation to generation. Obesity and its side effects are not conditions that you have to accept after they've been passed down from generation to generation. You can stop that legacy and model a better way for your children and those around you. You can say no to the bad eating habits and sedentary lifestyle that have become the norm in your family and community.

So many people in our society profit from the masses being fat and sick. Once you understand that, you can step outside the status quo and take back your freedom to live well. It won't be easy, but it will be worth it.

So, when I decided that I was going to make a change, I had to unlearn everything I had been taught about weight loss before. Remember, I had done the dieting thing many times before. My journey to almost four hundred pounds was not a straight line. I had yo-yo dieted and lost and gained weight many times along the way.

The problem was I had never figured out how our bodies work and what my body needed. The goals of health and fitness are generally universal, but everyone has their own approach for maintaining their health and fitness. Those who tout a new diet plan or workout tool as the solution for everyone's fitness woes are charlatans. I had to have some hard conversations with myself about my poor habits and the negative aspects of my lifestyle. I had to separate my mindset from that of even my familial culture. I had to decide that being comfortable was the enemy of my well-being.

I remember conversing with the surgeon who would later perform my hip replacement. He said that I would need to lose weight for the surgery and recovery to be successful. At almost four hundred pounds, you can imagine I had a way to go. So, in addition to extending my life, I knew that my mobility was at stake. I can only imagine what life would be like if I lost the ability to walk. That scared me, but it was also daunting.

There is pressure involved with knowing that you need to change your life but are at a loss for how to successfully make the change and not go back. I knew how to take two steps forward and three back, but I did not know how to lose weight and get healthy without ever going back. It took many conversations to strengthen my faith that I could do it. But you know what? I did it. I succeeded where my surgeon said only two others had, and those others were younger than me. I lost weight without any medical intervention, and I'm still walking and running strong. The best part is that my testimony is still growing!

I can do all things through Christ who strengthens me.
—Philippians 4:13

There comes a time when the excuses must cease, and the pedal must hit the metal. I had to look at myself in the mirror and remind myself that I could do anything I put my mind to. We all have the power to turn our situation around, and that extends past health and fitness into any area of life. Sometimes there are situations in life that affect us to the point that we neglect our self-care because they break our will to thrive. To do what needs to be done, you must deal with those issues. The health and fitness journey goes hand in hand with healing every part of yourself. There is no way I could have made the sacrifices I made every day and disciplined myself the way I needed if I was also dragging emotional and spiritual baggage around.

ANY CHANGE, EVEN A CHANGE FOR THE BETTER, IS ALWAYS ACCOMPANIED BY DISCOMFORTS.
—Arnold Bennett

Your body, mind, and soul need to rest and focus for real long-term changes to be achieved. Remember, this is a lifestyle change. There is no going back. Our bodies and minds want to return to what is familiar, so these changes will always need to be maintained and built upon. You will need to readjust when the things you once did don't work anymore. You will need to encourage yourself when you slip up to avoid staying there.

You see, these conversations were not just for the beginning of my health journey. I'm still having these conversations with myself. I had to have a few conversations with other people, too! My dear wife has always been supportive of me being my best. When I decided I was going to turn my health around, she was right there with me, doing everything she could to ensure my success. Part of that was meal prepping for me. She wanted to make sure that I always had healthy options available so that I was not tempted to eat something that would work against my ultimate goals. The only problem with that was that my upbringing kicked right in, and when I saw all the prepared food in the refrigerator, I felt pressure not to let it spoil and go to waste.

Remember that I grew up believing it's a cardinal sin to waste any amount of food. And don't get me wrong. I still don't like food going to waste, but that means I have to have conversations with myself and others about how much food is prepared and what portion sizes I need. Grocery shopping takes a little more planning and intentionality to buy what we need while avoiding food waste.

So, now my wife prepares food, vacuum seals it, and puts it in the freezer. That way, I always have healthy options, but I put less pressure on myself to eat it all quickly. The shelf life is extended. Things like that take honest conversations with yourself and others. You'll find that a bit of mirror checking, and communication goes a long way on this journey. Be real with yourself and others so you can win!

Be willing to talk to yourself with positivity and determination. Be willing to reject defeat and embrace the hard work. There is momentum-building power in failing, trying again, and succeeding. You are an overcomer, superstar! You must believe that to become the best version of yourself—the you that God created you to be.

Ultimately, I had to decide that I would never diet again. Just like I said at the very beginning of this book, there is no cookie-cutter recipe for the type of transformation I've experienced. My desire is to help you figure out what will work for you. You must be willing to get intimately acquainted with how your body thrives and responds to change. It will take time, patience, and many mental check-ins, but a few universal principles should help kick-start your journey.

We'll cover those in the next chapter.

What are you willing to give up to reach your health and fitness goals?

_____

_____

_____

_____

Who do you need to have conversations with for support on this journey?

_____

_____

_____

_____

What have you discovered that does not support your optimal health? What does work?

_____

_____

_____

_____

ADDITIONAL NOTES:

_____

_____

_____

_____

_____

_____

_____

_____

_____

_____

_____

_____

_____

THE ONLY THING IN YOUR WAY IS YOUR OWN MIND.

CHANGE YOUR THINKING!

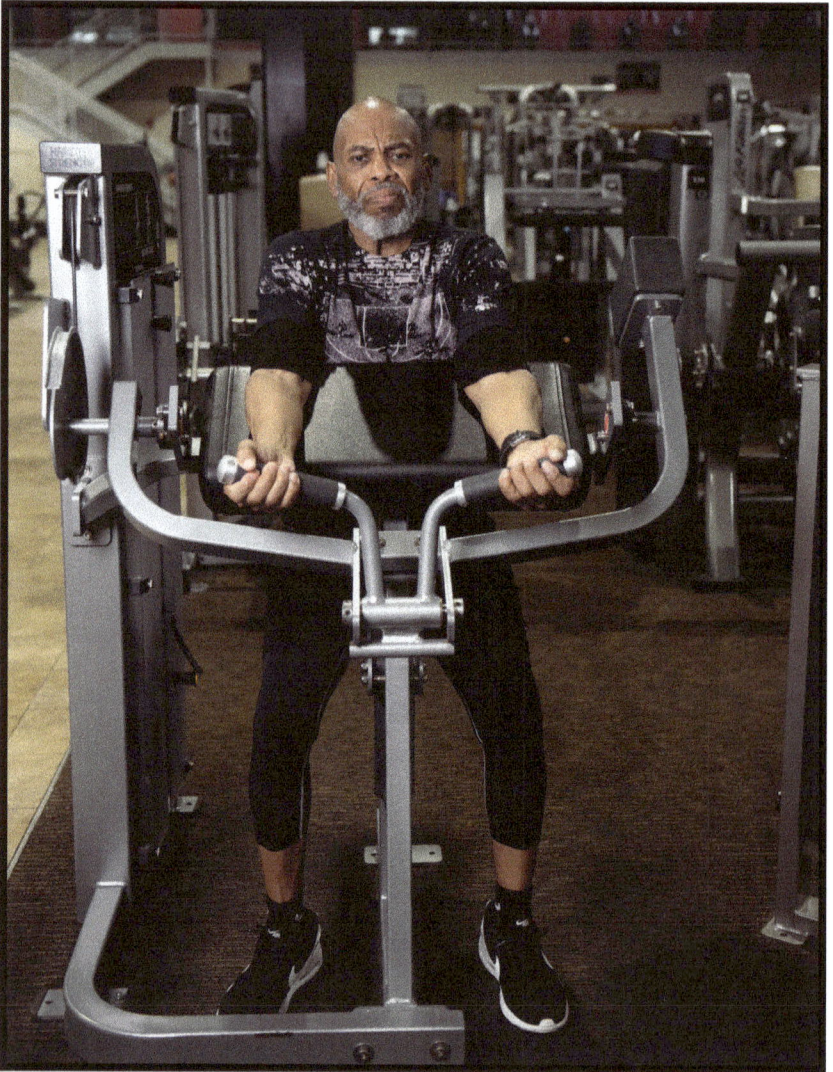

CHAPTER FIVE

THE JOURNEY

When I first see folks post weight loss, the question I get is "how did you do it? Many want a step-by-step plan so they can replicate my success, because no matter what size someone is, most people want to lose at least a few pounds these days. They want to know how long it took and what my specific diet plan was. My answer is always the same, though. What worked for me is not a one-size-fits-all solution.

The keys are that I changed how I eat, and I started being more active.

I went to a local gym, got a membership, and started going every day. I made space for caring for myself. I don't ascribe to a single diet plan. I just found aspects that work for me from several different ways of eating, and I found what dropped my pounds and gave me the nutrition I need to fuel my body and supply energy for me to move.

Some basic principles will work for everyone. The first is eating less. Fitness and nutrition professionals—which I am not—will often call this a caloric deficit. Calories are the universal unit of measurement for the fuel or energy value of any food we eat. Our body takes the calories we consume to fuel the functioning of our bodies.

So, on a fundamental level, if you eat more than your body needs on a regular basis, your body will gain weight because it needs to store those extra calories. Fat is the primary way that those extra calories are stored, and that excess fat causes all sorts of other processes to take place that can affect the way your body functions and how healthy you are.

So, a straightforward way to lose weight is to eat fewer calories than your body needs to function. It's simple—if you consume less than you need, your body will need to use the stored calories to run. When that happens, you'll lose weight. If you change nothing else about what you're eating and your activity level, you will lose weight just because you are eating less. It will take longer than any other method of weight loss, though, and if you're still eating junk, you will not heal your body.

My goal wasn't simply to lose weight, though! I wanted to get my body to optimal fitness and heal my body from the illnesses that my decisions had caused. For that, I needed to do more than just eat less of what I was already eating.

That brings me to the next basic principle: clean up the way you eat. I know this is not a popular step to take. These days, everyone is looking for a magic trick that will let you eat as much of what you like, but the truth is that we are only as healthy and fit as the fuel we put into our bodies. Think about luxury and high-performance vehicles. Many of them take a premium type of fuel, and the engines won't last as long or perform as well if any old fuel is used.

Our bodies are the same way. God put everything we need to live well on the earth when He created it, but we have come up with many ways to alter and process the goodness out of the food made to keep us healthy and whole. The adage "you are what you eat" is true. You can only function as well as what you put into your body.

The Standard American Diet, or SAD for short, is working against us. We have so many convenient processed options with added sugars and preservatives that are literally killing us. Most of us are on a high-fat, high-carbohydrate—otherwise known as sugar—diet.

So, on top of overeating, we are eating garbage. Many of the junk foods and processed foods that we consume lack the essential nutrients we need to live well. There are added chemicals that cause all sorts of problems in our bodies, and the calorie-to-nutrient ratio is abysmal. There is no way you will reach optimal health if you continue to eat the foods being sold to you on commercials and billboards.

To create a healthier diet for yourself, you must understand a few things about what comprises a well-balanced meal. Again, I won't get too deep into this, but you should have a daily diet where most of your calories come from fresh fruits and vegetables, whole grains, legumes, nuts, and lean proteins. Eating in this manner will provide you with all the daily nutrients

A HEALTHY OUTSIDE STARTS FROM THE INSIDE.

—Robert Urich

you need. The United States Department of Agriculture has dietary guidelines for Americans at health.gov, so check it out to learn more about what percentages you should eat of each category. The critical part is understanding that if you stay within these food groups and eat mainly whole foods—not processed—you will go a long way toward good health.

The last part of the equation is to exercise. Our bodies were designed to move dynamically! Now, this is the key that many folks try to use as a sole measure. They think that if they go to the gym six or seven days a week, they can get away with eating whatever they want. That's a lousy mentality because the truth is that you can look terrific on the outside and still be sick on the inside. You can't out-exercise a bad diet. They must work together if you want to reach optimal health.

So, along with cleaning up your diet and eating fewer calories, you will need to move your body. Now, this is going to look different from person to person. There are specific ways you can work out that will help to build muscle and help your body work more efficiently. In general, though, you can just start with simply walking for thirty minutes a day, and you'll likely see a significant improvement in your health and fitness.

The most important thing to remember is that this is a journey. You have to commit to the process of changing your mindset and life, then trust that the process is working even when you can't see huge results immediately. While every person's journey will look different, I want to share some snapshots from my journey so you know that you won't reach your goals overnight, but you can do it if you stay the course. I hope this peek into my journey helps kick-start your process of learning what works best for you, superstar!

Let's look at my journey after you think about the reflection questions below.

What specific dietary changes do you need to make for a healthier life?

_____

_____

_____

_____

How active are you currently? How can you move more going forward?

_____

_____

_____

_____

Evaluate your current diet. What foods can you cut out to eliminate empty calories (high-calorie foods that don't have much nutritional value)?

_____

_____

_____

_____

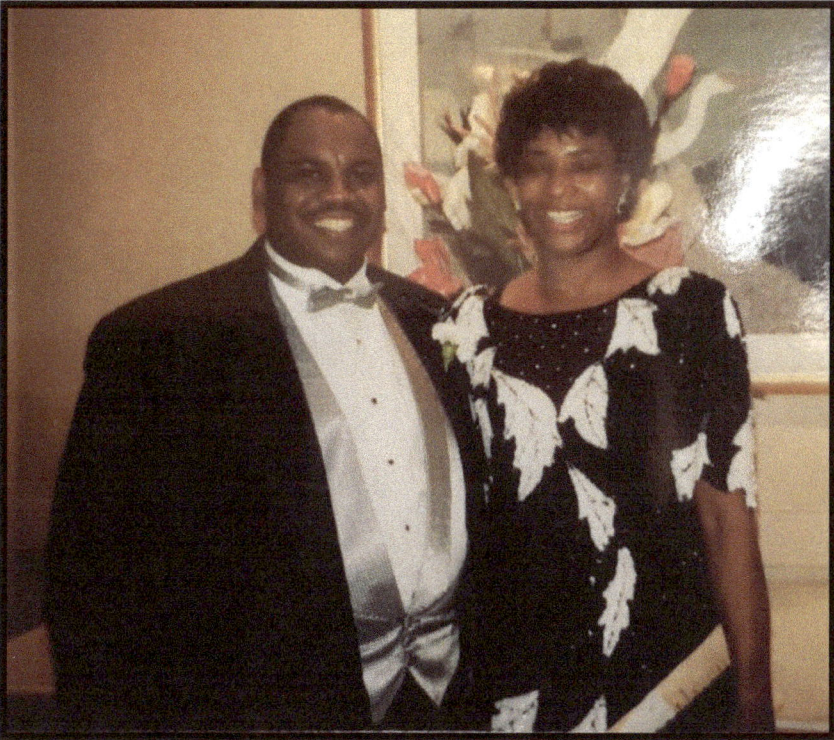

THIS IS BEFORE MY JOURNEY BEGAN.

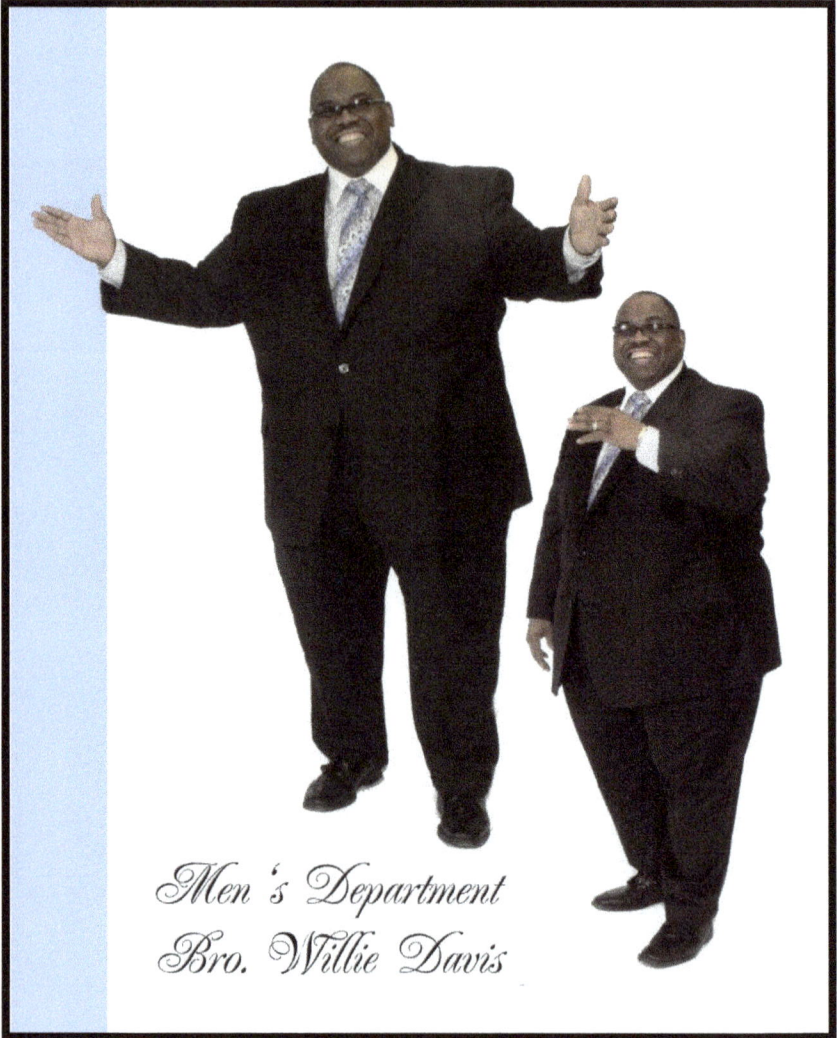

Men's Department
Bro. Willie Davis

I WAS STILL PUTTING EVERYTHING ELSE
BEFORE MY HEALTH AND FITNESS.

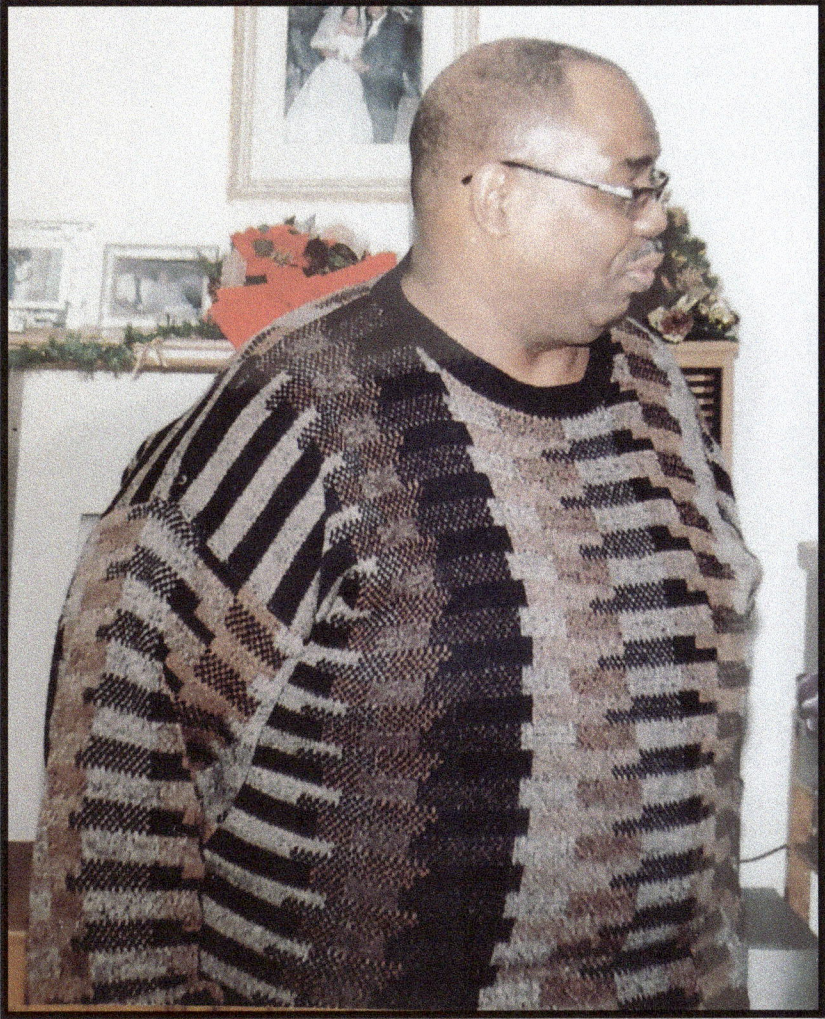

I STILL HAVE THIS SWEATER. DECENT LOOKING CLOTHES ARE EXPENSIVE WHEN YOU'RE BIG.

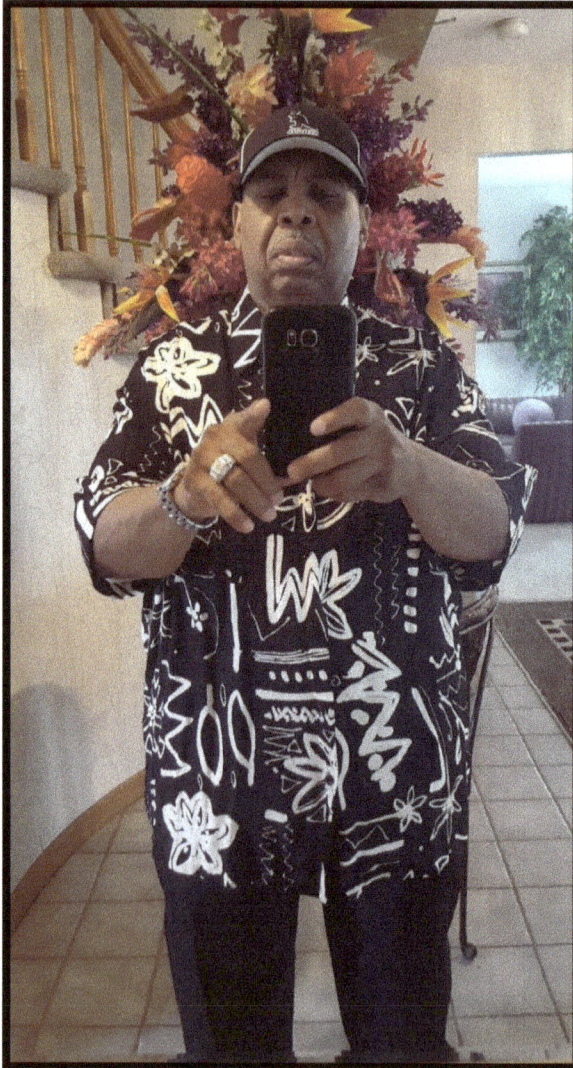

**SEEING RESULTS WAS GREAT MOTIVATION
TO KEEP GOING!**

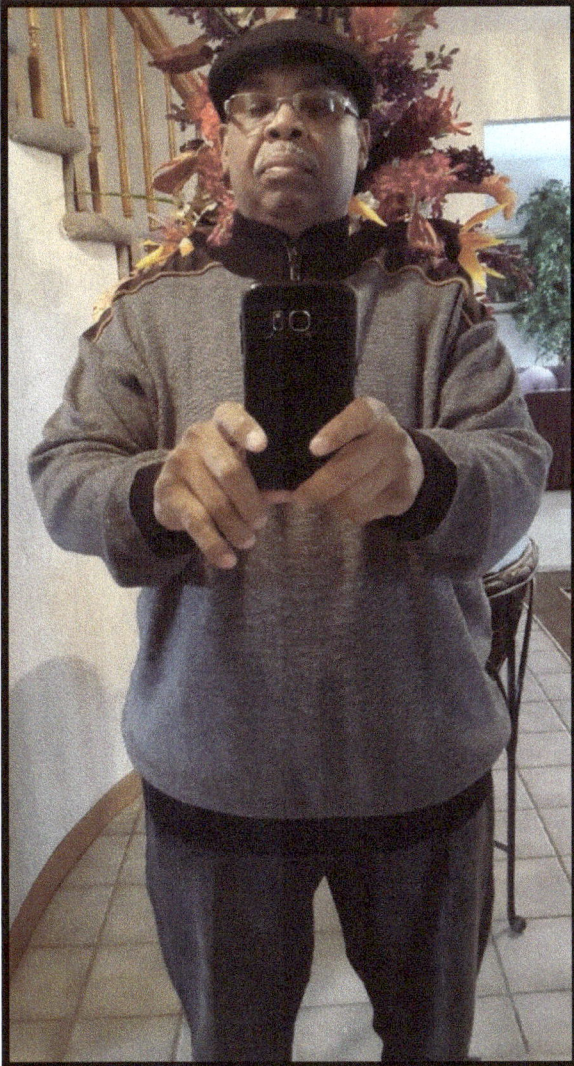

I WAS COMMITTED TO KEEP GOING.

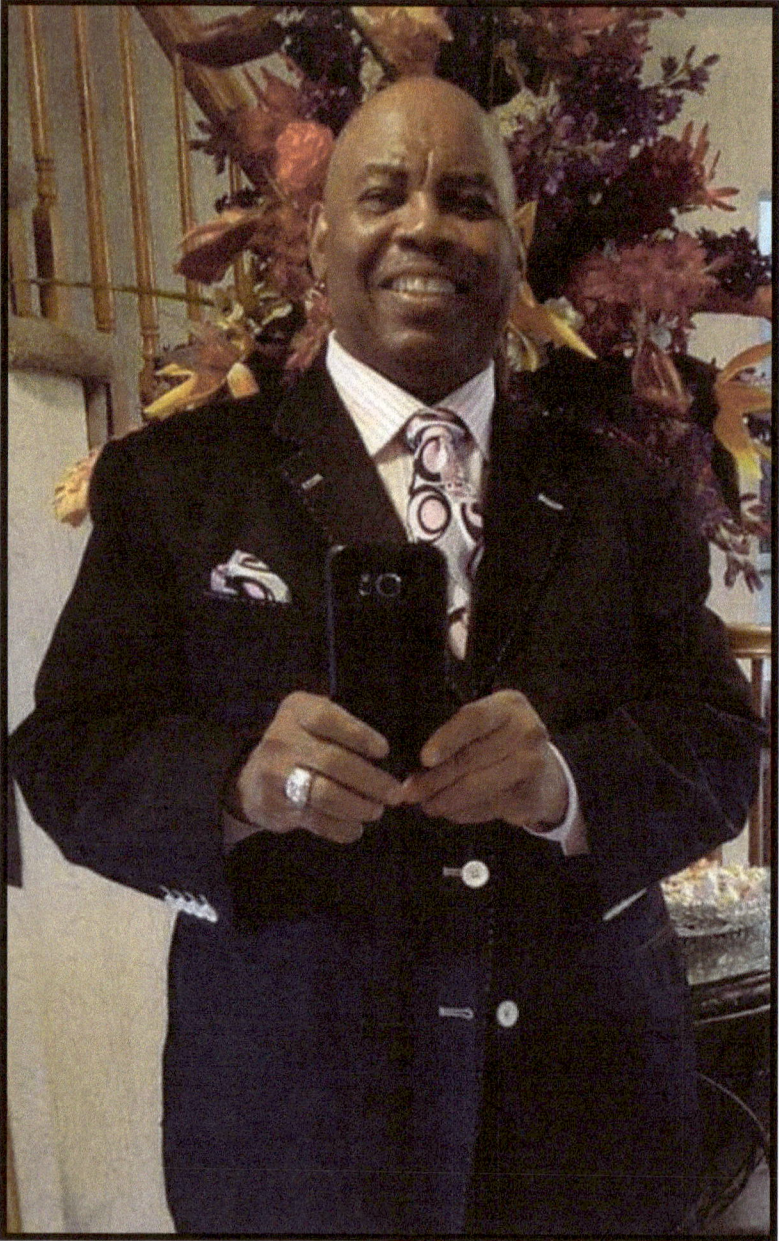

**FOLKS WERE IMPRESSED AT THIS POINT,
BUT I KNEW I STILL HAD WORK TO DO!**

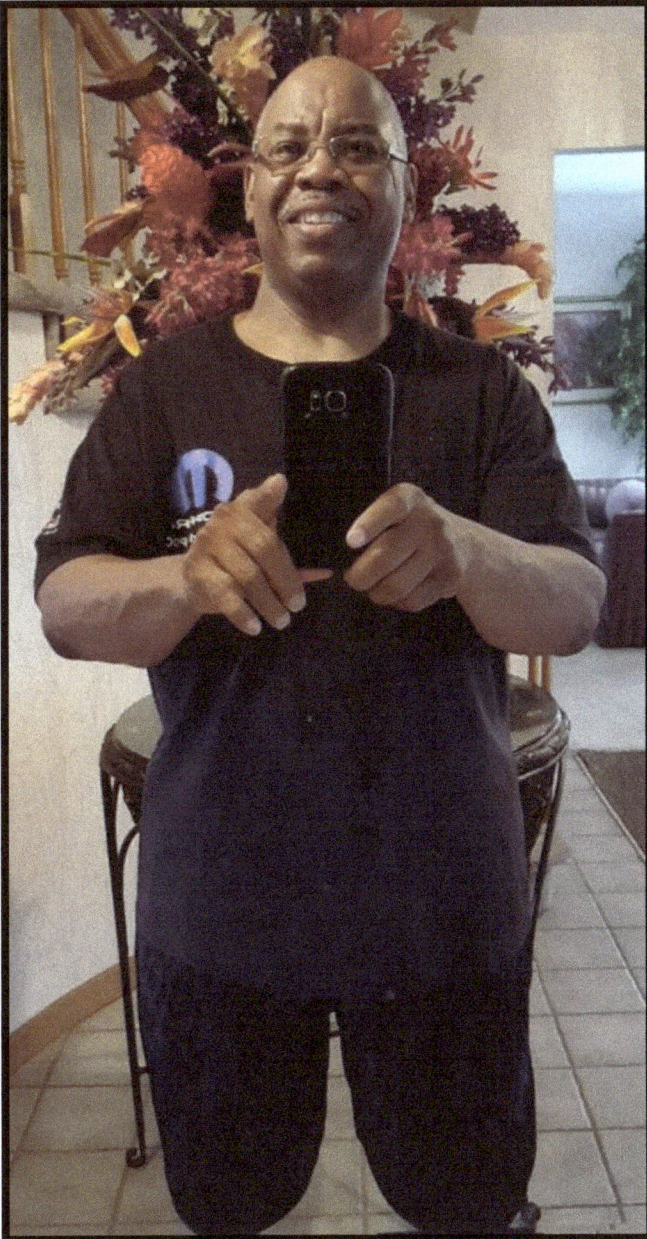

I WAS TRUSTING THE PROCESS!

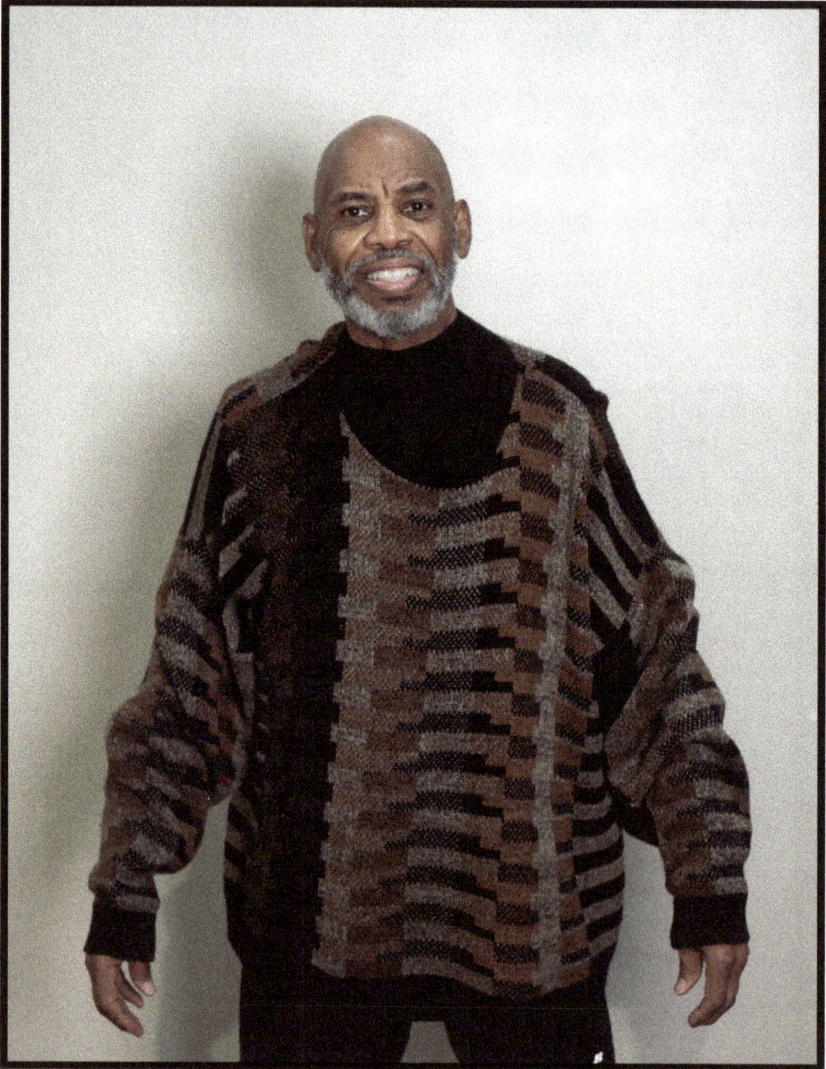

DO YOU REMEMBER THIS SWEATER?

YOU MUST LOSE THE OLD YOU TO FIND THE NEW YOU!

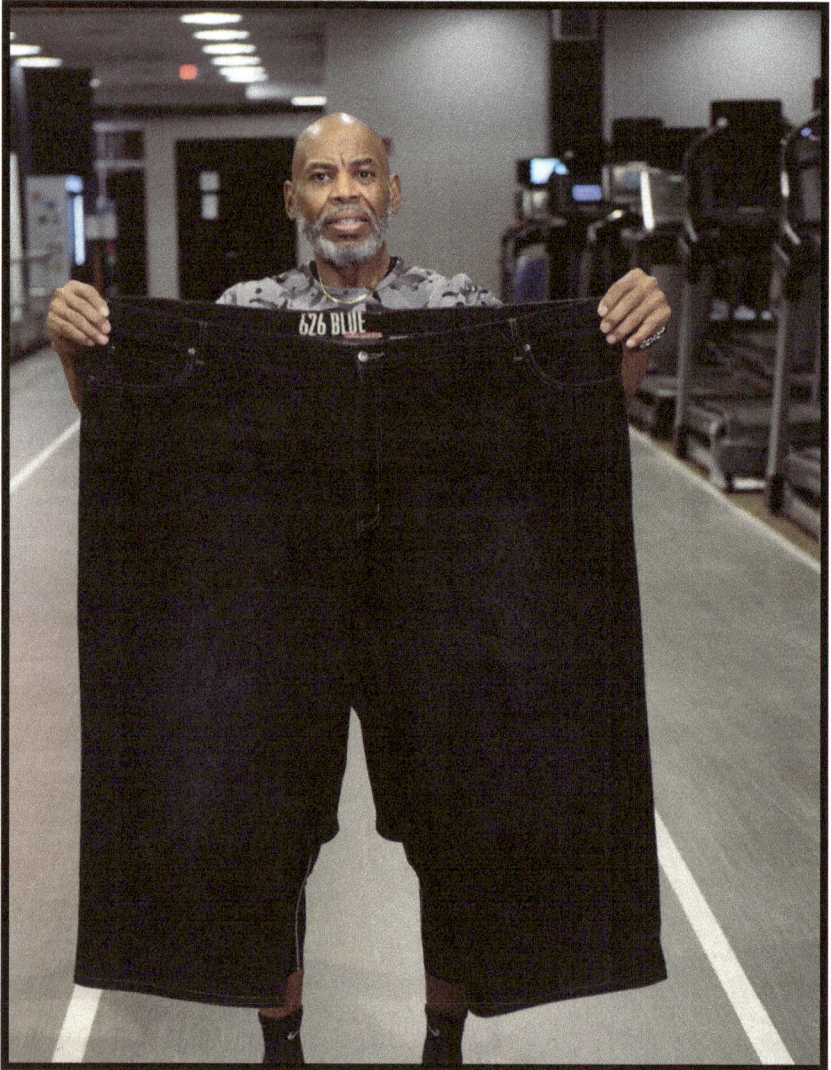

CHAPTER SIX

THE BRAND NEW ME

often marvel at how different my life is now. I have completely transformed my life in just a relatively short amount of time! My lifestyle and quality of life have been so much better since I decided to reclaim my health.

Since that first day, many events have enriched my life and the lives of countless others. I'm grateful for the opportunity to inspire so many people to do the hard work and get fit. One major improvement in my quality of life is the reversal of the illnesses I dealt with. The unfortunate truth is that both sides of my family had dealt with high blood pressure and obesity long before I came along.

Unfortunately, many of us just continued that tradition of poor health and have paid the price with our quality of life and, ultimately, our longevity. So, when I decided to get healthy, that legacy was one that I was determined to break. You don't have to accept poor health as an unavoidable consequence of familial genetics. You have everything you need to break free of those chains and start a legacy of optimal health in your family.

WHEN DIET IS WRONG, MEDICINE IS OF NO USE. WHEN DIET IS CORRECT, MEDICINE IS OF NO NEED.
—Ayurvedic proverb

For over ten months now, I have been completely off my medications! I'm not talking about a decrease in the dosage or frequency. I mean I don't have to take them anymore. For years I was on Lodipine for high blood pressure, and my cholesterol was 236 at one point. As I began making the changes that brought me to better health, I began to feel I didn't need the meds as much. So, about four days before one of my medical appointments, I stopped taking my blood pressure medications. I'm no medical professional, but I wanted my doctor to see my numbers without the medicine.

When I went to the appointment and shared what I'd done, my doctor informed me that I really needed to be off the medication for a few weeks before it was out of my system. He also shared that there is a proper way to wean off the medication. So, he cut my dose in half and said he would test me again. Three weeks before my next appointment, I stopped taking my medication altogether, and the labs came back great. So, he took me off the prescription for good.

There is no better feeling than getting rid of something that you thought would just be a lifelong issue. There is nothing like realizing that you have way more control over your health and quality of life than you previously thought. There is nothing like changing big and small aspects of your life and being able to maintain that change. Superstar, I am never going back to the way I was living! You don't have to look back either. I'm here to tell you that you have the power to move onward and upward! Aside from health, there are a bunch of benefits that can improve your quality of life.

For instance, there is nothing like being able to shop at any old store and have options in the whole rainbow of colors! You know, big folks get relegated to mostly dark colors like black, browns, and blues. So, there is nothing like being able to expand my color palette again. There is nothing like walking out of the bathroom with a towel tied around me that I don't have to hold to keep secure. There is no feeling like getting up and going with ease. There are so many benefits to getting healthy, and they aren't all physical. There is a mental release to not being self-conscious about my weight or how it affects my interaction with the world around me.

I was recently a part of a health program at the church I belonged to as a new Christian. The joy of participating and encouraging all the participants—young and old—was wonderful! We connected on a deeply spiritual level as we all pursued the quality of health that God created us to have.

Being able to walk miles at a time and have fun in the exercise classes was great! Frankly, once you make that decision, it does not matter if you have lost two hundred pounds or haven't lost a single pound yet; you have a bond with other people who are committed to getting healthy and fit. An affinity is born of the common goal to reclaim optimal health. I've made so many friends along the way, and we have great fun on this journey.

There are also new struggles. Along a weight loss journey, there are times that you plateau and must figure out what to change to keep moving in the right direction. You have to figure out what works for you long term and get comfortable with weight's natural ups and downs. Even once you hit your goal weight, you still must work to maintain your weight. It's normal to fluctuate within a five- to ten-pound range, and that's something that you just learn to recognize. I know now that if my clothing starts to get a little snug, I need to reevaluate and reel it in.

When you lose the type of weight that I've lost, it's almost like you must reacclimate yourself to the world. There are habits and measures that you're used to taking as an overweight member of society that no longer apply. It's exciting, but it can also take a while to relearn how to exist. When folks look at you in public, you must retrain your mind to not assume they are silently judging how much space you take up.

When you shop for clothing, you need to learn to free yourself from dark and forgiving items and enjoy looking good. People who have lost a lot of weight often deal with a kind of body dysmorphia that keeps them seeing a big person in the mirror, when in reality they look great! It is a long-term journey and struggle, but it's worth it!

It's exciting to see myself now and how far I've come. But I understand how hard it is to mentally and physically make this type of change, so I don't make this transformation lightly. I also don't take my responsibility to never go back lightly. I know how easy it is to slowly let yourself go. I know how quick we can be to fill our physical and figurative plates and look to convenience instead of the healthiest options.

I know how temporary pursuits can make us lose sight of our lifelong goals. I refuse to go back to the life I had. I love the brand-new me, and I'm looking to make it the brand new "we"! I believe in you, superstar. There is nothing you can't do if you put your mind and heart into it.

I've added years to my life. My grandchildren will get to have Grandpa Bill longer than before. I got to see my granddaughter graduate from college, buy her first condo, and host us for Thanksgiving while I was writing this book. There is a special kind of joy in seeing your legacy flourish right before your eyes. I will never again trade my years for an extra cheeseburger or slice of cake. Those days are over, and I see nothing but greater things ahead of me. I expect to sit at my grandchildren's weddings and witness great-grandchildren being born. I plan to share my story and watch others reclaim their years and legacy, too!

I will enjoy fullness in my later years, and you can do it too! God created each of us to do something specific before we leave here, and I intend to complete my assignment. The question is whether you have the capacity to complete your assignment. It takes energy, time, and vitality to live life well and enjoy it as intended.

Every decision you make that decreases your lifespan or diminishes your quality of life is a decision made to lower the chances of you accomplishing everything you can.

What are three things you want to accomplish before you die?

_____

_____

_____

_____

What change can you make starting today to get you one step closer to those accomplishments?

_____

_____

_____

_____

List the folks you'll enlist to keep you accountable:

_____

_____

_____

_____

ADDITIONAL NOTES:

ONCE YOU CHANGE YOUR LIFESTYLE, YOU'LL NEVER HAVE TO DIET AGAIN!

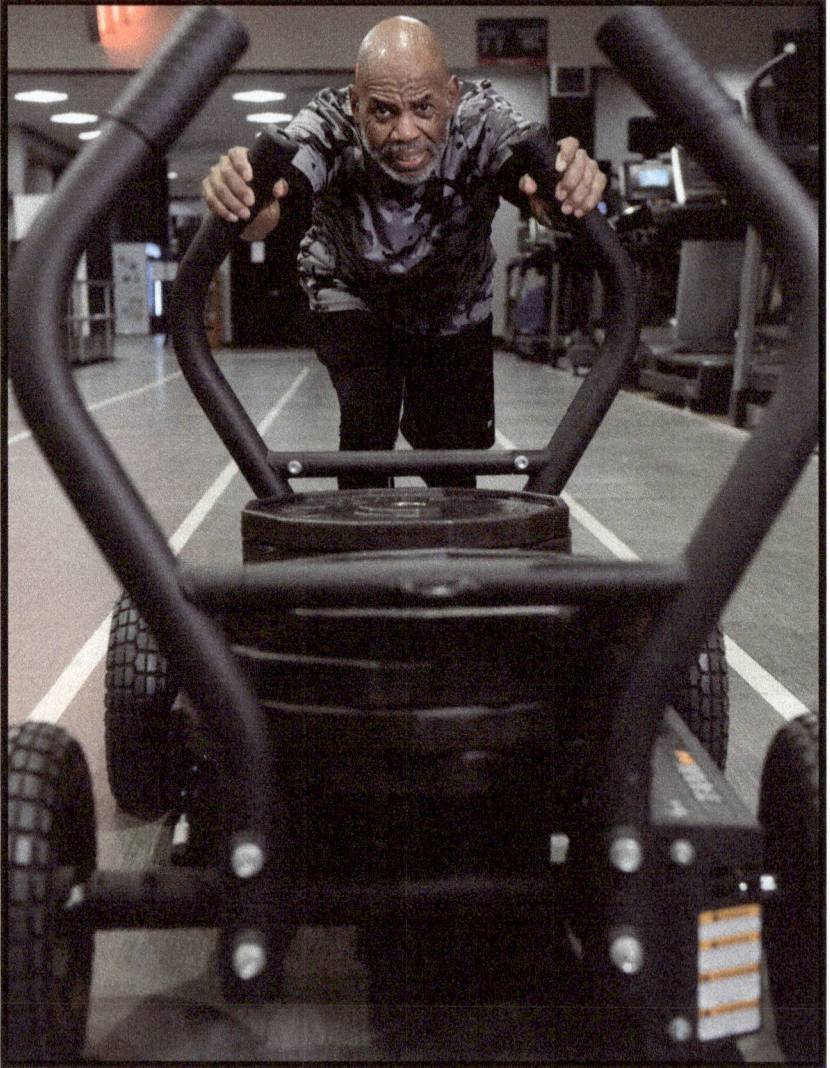

CHAPTER SEVEN

MOVING FORWARD

One of the lessons I've learned throughout this journey is that the journey never really ends, superstar! I can't stress this enough: this is not a diet or fitness plan—this is a lifestyle change! I still have food and fitness decisions to navigate daily. What makes it doable is that I've learned what works for me.

I've cultivated a new lifestyle and connected with a community of folks moving in the same direction. That's not to say that everyone in my circle fully understands and assists with the changes I've made, but I have been doing this consistently long enough to set a culture around myself. People know what to expect, and there are a lot of folks who are cheering me on and embarking on their own journey.

As I write this book, I am still embarking on new aspects of this new life. I have exciting projects and life events on the horizon. This book itself is something that I never thought would happen before I began this journey! A daily sense of excitement and expectation comes with moving into the lifestyle you're supposed to live. When you're fully living life, the sky is truly the limit!

It's not a cliché; it's a reality.

If you take nothing else from this, I want you to understand that there is no greater wealth you have than your health, and once you take control of that, you can do anything. I've found that my mindset has had to continually expand the deeper I got into this thing. I have had to face every harmful thought process that previously allowed me to stay unhealthy in order to maintain my current health. And, naturally, there will be old habits or thoughts that try to sneak back in from time to time, so I have to stay on top of my game.

I've also found that a key to my success was broadcasting my goals far and wide. I didn't embark on this journey in secret. It was important for me to gather a support system around me to cheer me on and keep me accountable. You will be surprised by who joins your cheer team on the journey to take back your health. As you take each step, the excitement will grow, and you'll build momentum.

This health and fitness part of my life has gone from being just a necessary measure to save my life to being a part of my daily life that brings me joy and power. I've found another kind of strength within myself that I'd never tapped into before, and it feels great!

To get this feeling, you must fully commit. There is no way to do it halfway and end up with similar results. This requires an all-or-nothing mindset!

It reminds me of being an athlete in my younger years. It wasn't enough to just practice offensive maneuvers and show up to the game. We had to have a good defense, as well. The same holds true in this health journey. I have to play the offense and defense, depending on the circumstance. When I'm at home, I can control what food is available and my activity options. When I'm traveling or at an event, I need to have practices in place to fall back on when what's available is not my preference.

A loose plan won't cut it. You really must take inventory, observe how your body works best, and develop a sustainable plan that you can execute under any number of circumstances.

It's a lot of work, but it has been worth it to add years back to my life. It's not just the time I've reclaimed, either; my present life is so much more enjoyable! Did you know that there is a gadget for just about every task that being obese makes difficult? There's a tool to help you put your socks on and a tool to help you expand standard seat belts. There are all sorts of extenders and stretchers. I no longer need to employ those methods to do everyday tasks, and I feel free!

The mentality of obesity has slowly been remodeled to the mindset of health and discipline. I no longer have the inner dialogues about food and the effort that simple tasks require. I no longer value convenience over quality. I no longer hold on to the habits of culture because that's what I was comfortable with.

Have you ever considered that comfort is the enemy of genuine change? There is a point at which you must decide that your comfort is not worth the years it's costing you. As I look forward, my only regret is that I didn't do this sooner. You have an immense opportunity before you, superstar; you can choose to change your entire life today! You don't even have to wait until the next moment. You can start this process right now!

There is no better time to truly begin to value yourself the way you were created to be valued. I know you've heard that your body is a temple, but many people don't grasp the depth of that statement. When you enter sacred spaces all around the world, there is a sense of reverence, peace, and calm. Your body should be that for you. You shouldn't have to feel like a prisoner inside your own body, bound by the choices you made yesterday that are affecting your tomorrow. You have the power to create a proverbial sanctuary inside yourself that provides that clarity and calm you need to take life by the horns and really live!

I'm looking to the future, and it is bright, superstar. All I want now is for you to join me in the light! It is a challenging journey, but the first step is easier than you'd think. Decide today, that you will not live another moment like you have in the past. Change the things you are consuming. That goes for the food you are physically consuming and much more. Change the conversations you allow yourself to have internally and the ones you have with others.

Change the books you're reading and the people you're following online. Feed your body, mind, and soul. Cultivate motivation, encouragement, and truth. You must believe that you're worth every fight it will take to create the new you.

You're worth it. I know it, but your life will never change until you believe it yourself.

ADDITIONAL NOTES:

YOU CAN DO THIS, SUPERSTAR!

GET TO WORK.

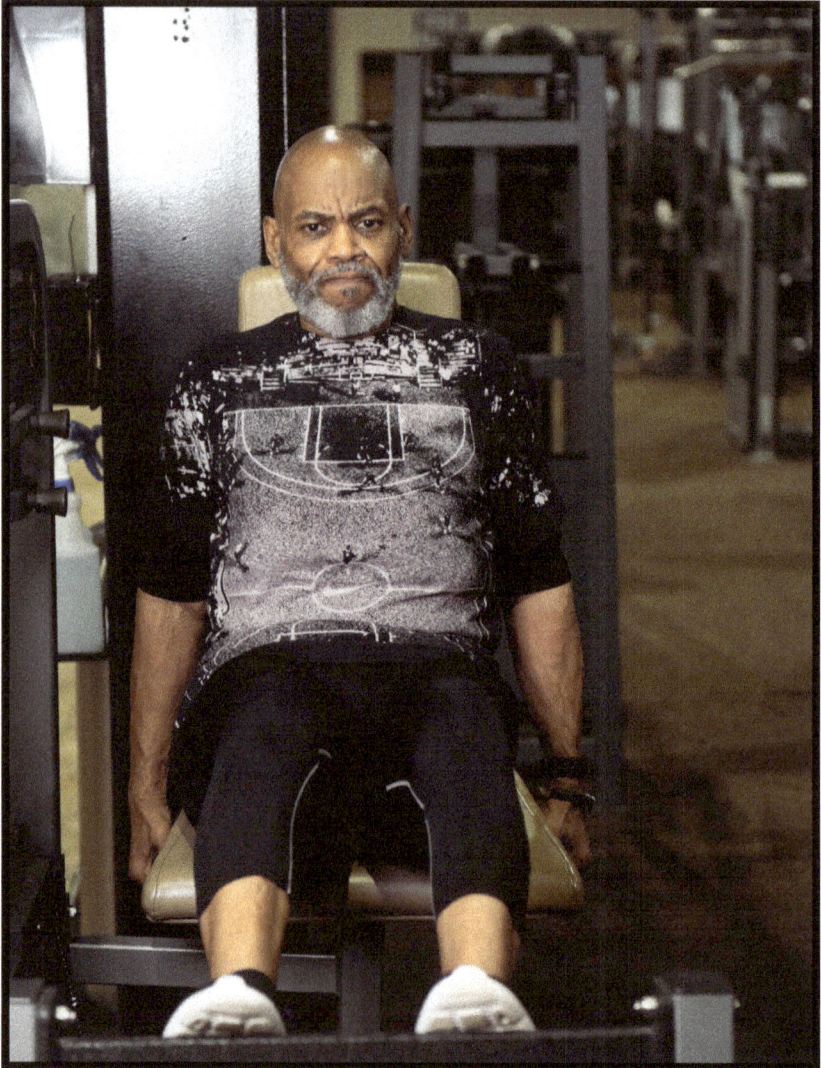

CONCLUSION

Thanks for sticking with me this long, superstar! I'm excited for you because I know that using the principles in this book and taking back control of your life will benefit you and others in ways that you can't even imagine. There is nothing you can't do when you make a decision and consistently choose to support that decision with your thoughts and actions.

As I reflect on the journey, the changes in my life, and even the lives of some people around me, I'm in awe. If you'd asked me five years ago whether I'd be where I am today, I probably would have laughed. Don't get me wrong; as I've mentioned before, I have tried many diets and plans over the years. But to be in a place where the weight and health issues are behind me, without dieting anymore, is a marvel.

I wake up each day with more certainty than the day before that I have started a new chapter in my story.

Before you put this book down and turn the page on your new chapter, I want to leave you with a few thoughts to help get you started!

Plan and prepare.

You must make your vision clear and commit to it within yourself as you start this journey. Now, this doesn't have to be an intricate plan, but just a clear focus on why you're doing this, committing to a "no excuse" mentality, and taking a little time to think about how you need to restructure your lifestyle to succeed. This may mean getting up a little earlier to exercise or planning meals each week so that you aren't tempted to fall back on the same eating habits from before.

Be kind to yourself.

You are embarking on a seriously challenging journey. It will take time, consistency, and perseverance. It's a given that you'll get tired and want to give up. You will consider having that extra-large slice of cake. You will be invited to social events where the menu leaves you with few options that fit into your new lifestyle. Be kind to yourself in those challenging moments of temptation, but don't give up! You are more than a conqueror, superstar! That doesn't mean there will be no battle. It means you will win the war!

Get ready to celebrate you!

Once you've decided to value your health and wellness enough to commit to changing your life, you should be dedicated to celebrating every bit of progress and success. Give yourself a pat on the back when you control your portions or lose a single pound. In the beginning, especially, the triumphs may seem small or far between.

There may be naysayers or the ever-present "other" to compare yourself to. Resist that urge. You are doing the best things you could be doing for yourself and your legacy, so get ready to affirm yourself with every step you take forward. And know that I'm celebrating you too!

Remember that this is a new lifestyle.

You've heard it many times. I've said it a bunch of times in this book alone. Forget the diets and quick-fix fitness programs. This is a journey that will span the rest of your life. So, you need to figure out the sustainable lifestyle choices you can make to maintain the wealth of your health. It's not sustainable to deprive yourself of every culinary pleasure for the rest of your life, but it is possible to reshape the way you eat for good. Things like portion control and cleaning up your overall eating habits will work wonders.

The adage that too much of a good thing can be bad is true. So, just remember this one word: moderation. Living life in moderation will work wonders for everything from your pants size to your spiritual health.

Start today!

If you haven't already decided to start this journey, do it now. Don't wait until tomorrow, Monday, or the first of the month. You can start right this minute. Flip that mental switch that tells you that you have to figure it all out before you begin. Take a few minutes now to decide and commit to the change, and you'll be on your way to success. Today is the first day of the rest of your life, so make it count! Every second that you make better decisions is a second of your life reclaimed.

You can start to lengthen your life starting now. You are going to be adjusting and making changes as you go because you'll find that your body may respond differently than those around you. That's okay! You must learn what works for you, and the sooner you start, the sooner you'll hit your goal.

There will be folks around you who share what worked for them and what they think is best. While it's true that some universal principles work for most (see chapter 5), there is no one-size-fits-all plan for success. You must be willing to drown out the noise around you and listen to your body.

Staying in tune with what is working for you and what isn't working for you will help you become healthy sooner. Find recipes that incorporate the right foods and appeal to your tastes. Try different exercises and find the complete plan that you can enjoy while getting results. The main thing is to figure out what you will continue to do instead of forcing yourself to use methods that you can't maintain because they make you miserable.

It will be hard, but this journey can bring you joy. So, lean into that superstar; the best is yet to come. Saving Grandpa Bill is much bigger than just me. It's about bringing everyone along with me that I can!

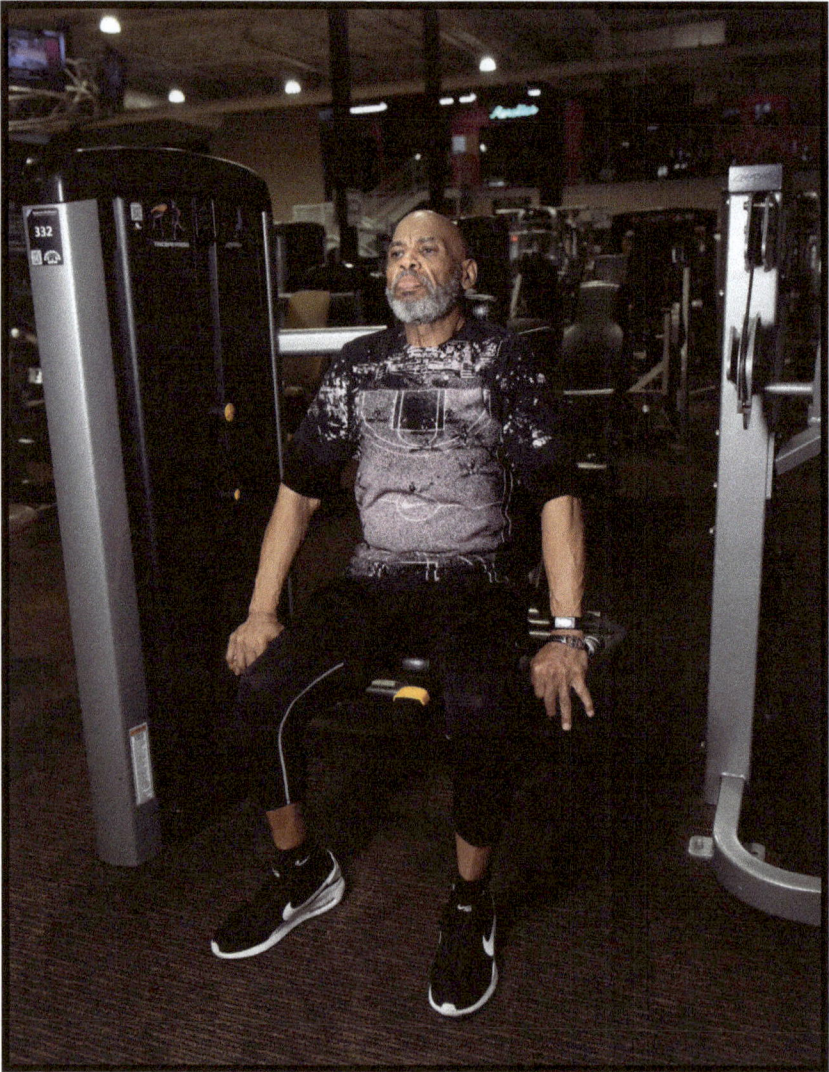

Pedaling towards The Brand New Me
one day at a time.

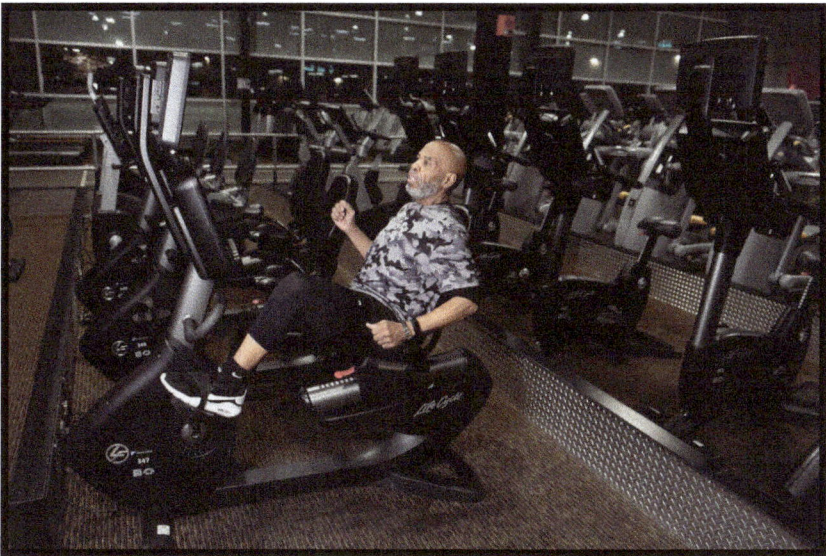

The Life Fitness Life Cycle isn't just a piece of exercise equipment; it's been my steadfast companion on this journey of transformation.

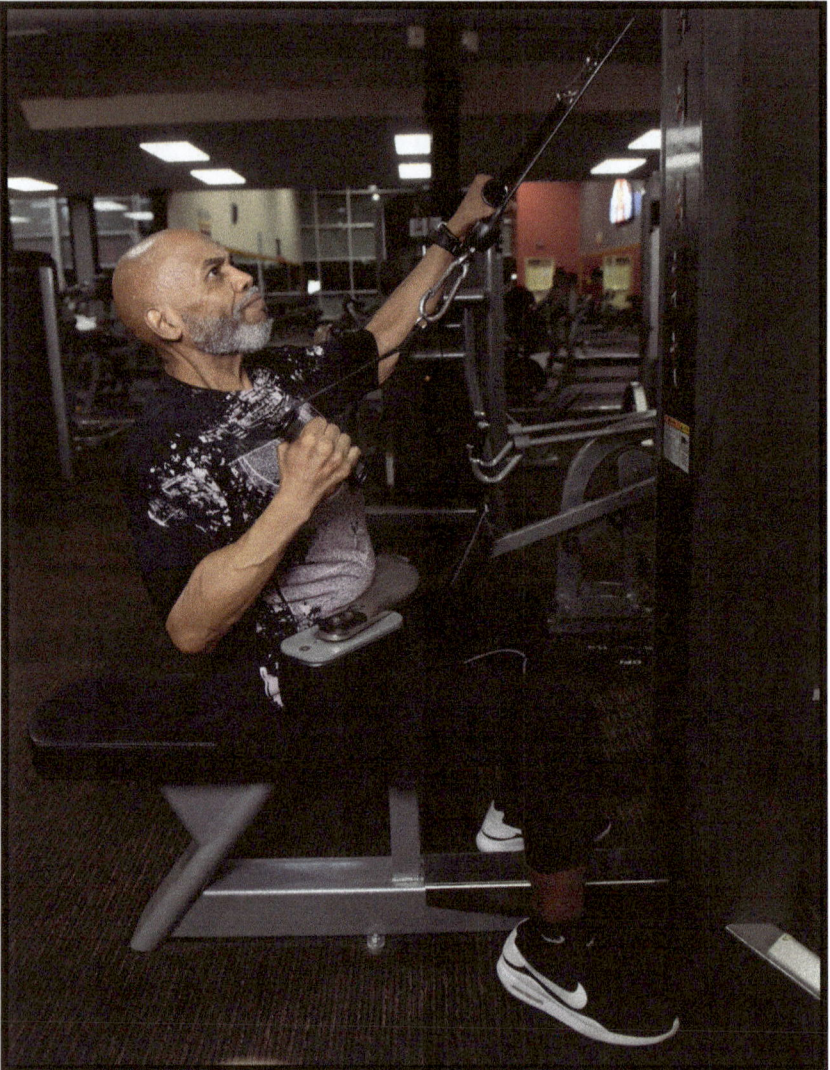

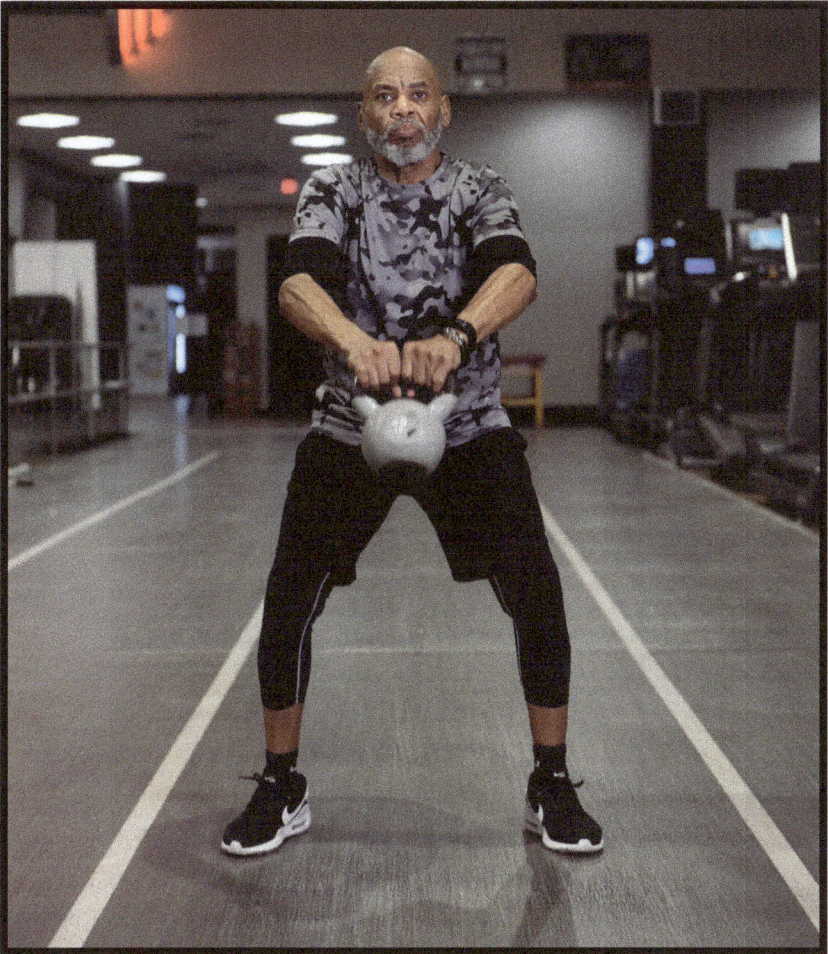

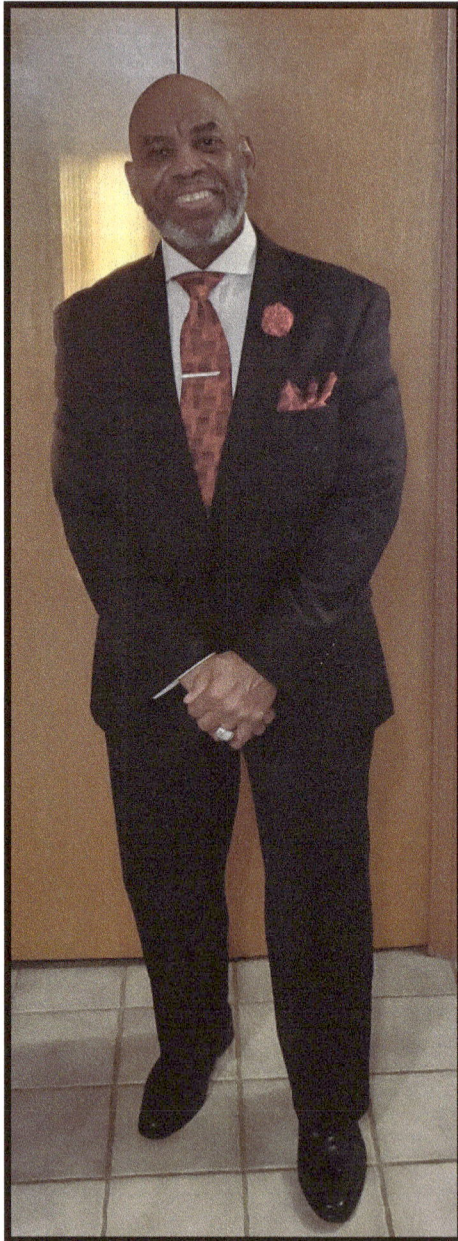

ABOUT THE AUTHOR

Willie "Bill" Davis is not just an author; he's a CEO, visionary thinker and a devoted family man. With an enduring 43-year marriage to his wife Denise, five cherished children, and eleven adored grandchildren, Bill's life has been profoundly enriched by the love and wisdom of his extended family and friends. His journey into retirement began in 2009 after a dedicated 35-year career at Chrysler Corporation, where he worked tirelessly and ascended to the role of a clerk/team leader. This professional journey not only honed his work ethic but also instilled in him valuable lessons about teamwork, resilience, and unwavering commitment..

However, what truly sets Bill apart is his extraordinary personal transformation. At the age of 66 1/2, he embarked on a remarkable weight loss journey that defied all odds, shedding a remarkable 225 pounds in just 22 months—without resorting to surgeries, procedures, medical diet plans, pills, or trainers. Today, he stands at a healthy and lean 150 pounds, maintaining this incredible weight loss for over 20 months. This awe-inspiring fitness and health transformation is a central theme in his work, intricately woven with his dedication to family, community, church, and personal growth.

For more information about Willie, The Brand New Me, LLC and the incredible journey that defines his life, visit:

www.williebilldavis.com

www.ingramcontent.com/pod-product-compliance
Lightning Source LLC
Chambersburg PA
CBHW052118030426
42335CB00025B/3032